For William, Robert and Alison

Nursing Power and Social Judgement

MARTIN JOHNSON, RN, MSc, PhD
Professor of Nursing
University of Central Lancashire
Preston

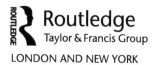
Routledge
Taylor & Francis Group

LONDON AND NEW YORK

First published 1997 by Ashgate Publishing

Reissued 2018 by Routledge
2 Park Square, Milton Park, Abingdon, Oxon OX14 4RN
711 Third Avenue, New York, NY 10017, USA

Routledge is an imprint of the Taylor & Francis Group, an informa business

Publisher's Note
The publisher has gone to great lengths to ensure the quality of this reprint but points out that some imperfections in the original copies may be apparent.

Disclaimer
The publisher has made every effort to trace copyright holders and welcomes correspondence from those they have been unable to contact.

A Library of Congress record exists under LC control number: 97071457

ISBN 13: 978-1-138-33075-7 (hbk)
ISBN 13: 978-1-138-33076-4 (pbk)
ISBN 13: 978-0-429-44766-2 (ebk)

Contents

Tables

Introduction

This book is about the judgemental labelling of people in hospital care. Despite its focus of data collection being one medical ward, the issues it raises doubtless have significance for most health and other professions who have responsibility for achieving compliance with medical or social goals. Previously described by Stockwell (1972), Fielding (1986) and others, being seen as good, bad, popular or unpopular has been commonly seen as a concomitant of certain traits or characteristics which individuals possess, such as being elderly or having a certain type of illness such as stroke.

The field work was done in the warm summer months when I voluntarily worked as a bank staff nurse but also presented myself openly as a researcher. I did follow-up interviews over the succeeding months. I worked as a nurse in the ward and utilised an ethnographic approach in which overt participant observation and conversational interviews were important sources of data. Themes emerged during the analysis which refute the traits theory of social judgement (or moral evaluation) which is implicit in most previous work.

I describe the phenomenon of social judgement in some detail and set it into a discussion of the social context where an unequal balance of power is integral to provider-recipient relationships. Here it becomes clear that a relationship exists between the need for nurses to sustain their power over patients and the use of labels as part of this process of disempowerment. Judgemental labelling is seen from an interactionist perspective as a process through which care is managed and which provides nurses with a strategy for coping with the emotional labour of care. For descriptive purposes the process is analysed in four categories, of judging people, negotiating, struggling and acquiescing. Categories of caring and coping are discussed as an illustration of some of the potential consequences of caring in a climate of judgemental labelling. Of particular interest were categories of excellent care which nurses provided, sometimes covertly, as apparent compensation for the perceived deleterious effects of negative social evaluations of patients. In other situations we used coercive and paternalistic approaches which open the door to morally questionable conduct.

I conclude the book with a summary of the beginning (or substantive) theory of social judgement as it was evident to me in Howarth ward at a large city teaching hospital. I challenge the common conception of consensus upon and permanence of labels, since ideas of negotiation and conflict were very necessary to my understanding and interpretation of the data as it emerged. I make a number of provisional recommendations such as that nurse researchers and educators should do more clinical research and attempt to utilise more participatory and action-oriented methods in the future. I further suggest that attention to the micropolitics of the patient-care relationship is very important to the understanding of moral questions in health care where decisions are clearly made in relation the context rather than textbook principles. Currently this context is laden with subjective evaluations of social value of persons, a vital consideration in moral decision-making.

I am indebted to a large number of people who in various ways have enabled me to undertake this study, the substance of which was presented for a PhD of the University of Manchester. Professor Christine Webb combines the rare qualities of exceptional clarity of thought, attention to detail and sensitivity when my work needed substantial revision. Having a realistic appreciation of my other lives, since I was a part time student, she also knew just when to give me a nudge to get back on target and was an immense source of support. In course of the work I attended Professor John Harris's health care ethics lectures. As the work developed it became one more of applied sociology of health care than of moral philosophy. He nevertheless maintained an interest and has been the source of some key challenges to my previously rather orthodox thinking about nursing and moral issues. My debt to Alison, William and Robert Johnson who made great sacrifices enabling the work to be completed, is great indeed.

The nurses and patients on Howarth ward bore my intrusion into their world without complaint and I thank them dearly for their time and kindness. If any portion of this work could be construed as a criticism of them as individuals then I have misrepresented the argument. Rather, I seek to describe nursing as both I and they practiced it in Howarth ward for those few months. Both grumbling and brilliant care were facts as I saw them, and are strategies for dealing with what would otherwise be impossible strain.

Martin Johnson, July 1997

1 Research perspective

A good deal has been written about research perspectives in qualitative research (Schwartz and Jacobs, 1979; Silverman, 1975; Denzin,1992). Various approaches have been identified, and much debate takes place about definition and emphasis of particular traditions. For example, the terms phenomenology, symbolic interactionism, ethnography, feminist methodology and even ethnomethodology seem to be used frequently and with a good degree of overlap. What can be said with some degree of confidence is that these approaches together constitute a reaction to, if not an attack upon, the cultural and scientific dominance of positivism, particularly in Europe, America and more recently Australasia.

Positivism

Positivism can be seen as the belief that both natural and social phenomena can, given the right developments in methods of classification and measurement, be recorded as facts. That is to say that there is assumed to be an 'objective reality' which can be identified, and which persists (Hammersley, 1992). Generally speaking positivist methods involve the production of 'hypotheses' which the method sets out to verify or refute. These hypotheses are often (though this is not always stated) deduced from extant theory in the social, behavioural or biological sciences (see for example Boore, 1978). Every attempt is made within the positivist tradition to remain 'value free', or neutral, and any attempt to record mediating social processes or meanings may be seen as inappropriate. Writing as ethnographers but in order to give some flavour of what this can mean for the observation of the social world, Hammersley and Atkinson (1983:4) suggest that:

> Scientific theories must be founded upon - tested by appeal to - descriptions that simply correspond to the state of the world, involving no theoretical assumptions and thus being beyond doubt. This foundation could be sense data, as in traditional empiricism, or as with

later versions, the realm of the 'publicly observable': the movement of physical objects, such as mercury in a thermometer, which can be easily agreed upon by all observers. Because observation in the social world is rarely as straightforward as reading a thermometer, this concern with a theoretically neutral observation language has led to great emphasis being given to the standardisation of procedures of observation. (Hammersley and Atkinson, 1983)

Among the many accounts of the arguments against such a position for social scientists, the most detailed exposition I have encountered is that of Denzin (1992). Drawing upon a rich historical account of the ideological and intellectual influences on qualitative researchers, Denzin explains some otherwise subtle differences between the various schools of interpretive sociology and their reaction to positivism. Hammersley and Atkinson (1983) explain the general thesis by arguing that non-positivists claim that the social world cannot be understood in terms of causal relationships or universal laws. This, they suggest is because human actions are based upon, or 'infused by', social meanings such as attitudes, motives, intentions and beliefs. They give as their example the assumption in much positivist social research that a stimulus-response model explains social behaviour without considering mediating processes. In the view of interactionists and other non-positivists:

> ...people interpret stimuli, and these interpretations, continually under revision as events unfold, shape their actions. (Hammersley and Atkinson, 1983:7)

Hammersley and Atkinson continue with the suggestion that stimuli can mean different things to different people and indeed to the same person at different times. This point is one of those crucial to the understanding of what I take to mean the interactionist perspective, and it turns out to be central in the understanding of the social process of evaluation or judgement of character in the context I describe.

Are qualitative and quantitative complementary?

There has been a good deal of argument concerning the merits of qualitative and quantitative research, and some views seem to be in favour of some sort of reconciliation (Leininger, 1985; Corner, 1991). For some time it was fair to say that feminist methods were broadly allied to the qualitative domain. Reinharz (1992) extensively documents this situation but concedes that in the post-modern era there may be strategic if not empirical benefit in multi-method research drawing upon both the main paradigms. Recent studies claiming a feminist perspective (see

4

Smith, 1992) combine both approaches in some degree although sometimes the mixture can seem ill-matched. I am, however, left with a sense of unease that the two paradigms involve such substantial difference of beliefs about the nature of knowledge and the conduct of research that the nature of their compatibility requires a good deal of clarification if they can co-exist at all sensibly in the same study.

Symbolic interactionism

In this project, both in the early phase in which I produced discussion papers on method and some epistemological concerns (Johnson, 1990, 1992), and more recently during data collection and analysis, I have inevitably drawn guidance from a range of viewpoints on research perspective. The most influential of these is probably what I would broadly term symbolic interactionism and specifically the Straussian 'negotiated order' perspective.

According to Denzin (1992), who has been an influential worker in this tradition for many years, interactionism grew largely from the influence of anthropology and phenomenology in the 1920's in the USA. Many of what later became known as the *Chicago School* of sociologists were, however, either European émigrés or of that extraction. Denzin's detailed history gives a good deal of importance to those writers such as Goffman (1959) and Strauss (see Glaser and Strauss, 1967) who consistently set out to refute the verificationist (positivist) position which was dominant in sociology at that time. Goffman's dramaturgical model, taking many of its constructs explicitly from a conception of social life as acting or drama, threw a fascinating light on the otherwise mundane and commonplace. It is impossible, as can be seen from my account of my experiences in Howarth ward, not to draw considerable insight from his work. Goffman's notions of *moral career* and *inmate* have a special relevance to my own discoveries, even when analysed through contemporary eyes.

As to the late Anselm Strauss (he died in 1996), his influence has been immense. He and Barney Glaser developed the now widely used analytic approach of grounded theory which is based firmly in assumptions about the value of an interpretive approach to human action (Glaser and Strauss, 1967). Theory generated by this method tends to emphasise processes rather than causes or outcomes although these latter help to expand the theory. Denzin (1992) suggests that Strauss's conception of interactionism stresses indeterminacy and danger in everyday life. Here the concept of negotiation comes into its own as a frame of reference for the discussion of all social processes. It makes explicit the notion that no social phenomenon is permanent or wholly determined by specific traits or variables. This seems eminently plausible. Indeed despite awareness of many limitations of my own analysis I remain concerned at the degree to which investigators claim to have utilised interactionist insights and methods such as grounded theory, but have clearly failed to grasp this fundamental point of negotiated social order which is integral to the approach (examples are Lorber, 1975; Stockwell, 1972 and Wilkinson 1991 whose work I examine in some detail later).

Without wishing to exalt either individuals or their work, especially when they themselves deprecate that trait among their opponents the positivists (see Glaser and Strauss, 1967), the extent to which I draw upon the work of Strauss and a large number of his colleagues will become clear over the course of this thesis. To the extent that an interactionist perspective does then inform and guide my method and my analysis.

Phenomenology and other perspectives

Among many differences of interpretation, three clear positions upon what phenomenology is stand in relation to the rest. On the one hand some American writers such as Lynch-Sauer (1985) see phenomenology as a specific method of qualitative research which contrasts with grounded theory or ethnography. She argues that the phenomenological method attempts to describe the specific 'lived experiences' of individuals with a minimum of interpretation by the researcher. Benner (1984), whose work is immensely influential, suggests another version of phenomenology which allows of more interpretation by the researcher. She claims that her analysis of nurse's progression from novice to expert status was drawn out using an approach she says derives from Martin Heidegger, but recently these claims have drawn substantial criticism. Cash (1995) for example, argues that Benner's basic Dreyfus and Dreyfus (novice to expert) framework pre-existed the investigation and that Benner has merely fitted her data into it. Perhaps more serious is the sustained attack by Crotty (1996) in which he shows that Benner and her followers have failed to grasp the fundamental tenet of phenomenology: that it is *phenomena* rather than 'subjective lived experience' or 'narrative' which should be the main object of investigation.

It is not my wish to sustain confusion in these matters, but I think, however, that yet a third position has much to commend it. Among ethnographers such as Bogdan and Taylor (1975) and more recently Hammersley and Atkinson (1983) the most consistent position adopted is that phenomenology represents the paradigm, or large domain in which other non-positivist approaches lie. It is a convenient opposite to positivism, one which, broadly speaking, accepts multiple definitions of social reality with which social scientists in general and nurses in particular are mostly concerned. My study therefore, could be defined as phenomenological. This would, however, give no real indication of the types of concepts I am likely to find useful, or indeed of the method I am likely to use to collect and analyse my data.

Other perspectives with which I would claim to be associated would be the following. First, there is an important choice to be made in how data are not only to be collected but also written up. Amazingly, some accounts of this type of phenomenological or naturalistic research are still written in the 'objective' style of the third person singular. As Webb (1992) argues, this is inconsistent with any acknowledgement that the researcher is both present and has an unavoidable effect upon the setting. It is therefore more honest, Webb argues, if the presence of the researcher in the setting is explicit and when the appropriate mode of writing is used. This is not a minor point, since language (broadly defined) is a very powerful, if not the only, method through which meanings are shared in the social world. This point of Webb's is amply supported by Porter (1993). It is, as Webb (1992) observes, only in nursing literature that a pseudo-objectivity has been required in some of the academic journals and even then not consistently so. Indeed she argues further that even in positivistic studies to write as if the researcher had no human part to play in proceedings is misconceived and could even be seen as deceptive.

Reflexivity

Reflexivity is seen by Steier (1991) as "a turning back of one's experience upon oneself". I attempt in this book to illustrate my reflexivity by discussing my perceptions of my participation in the setting. Of course the inclusion of myself as a participant makes the research semi-autobiographical. Some passages are highly personal, and whilst this can seem self-indulgent, with an appropriate balance it can represent researcher integrity and awareness. Such is for the reader to judge, but at least there is no attempt to conceal my effect on the setting even if I am unable to describe it accurately or in its entirety.

Hammersley (1990) identifies several modes of writing which appear in varying balance in qualitative research. Naturalism is that in which pure description occurs with relevant theory. Legitimatory mode is like this section, in which purpose and methods are explained. Confessional mode is the 'inside story' in which an inappropriate balance can seem too journalistic or indulgent. Such matters may also be aesthetic and so experimentation may be necessary. I believe that I utilise at least these three modes of writing, and that the humanistic orientation of my research perspective should be evident from the text. Reflexivity involves an awareness by an investigator of the degree to which they are making their own interpretation of events which might, indeed inevitably, would be portrayed otherwise by other writers. It involves reflecting constantly upon events as they unfold, and responding by following up notions which emerge as important in fieldwork rather than from preliminary reading.

Ethnography

I define ethnography, following Hammersley and Atkinson (1983), very broadly indeed. It consists of study of the social life, social world, or other aspects of the culture of a particular group or social setting. The methods and perspectives are commonly qualitative and phenomenological but not exclusively so. The word does however commonly assume a 'participant observation' approach, although as I outline later some investigators (although I am disinclined to agree with them) are prepared to classify interviews as a form of participant observation. Ethnography then, constitutes both a method (mainly involving fieldwork) and could also be said to be a perspective. In using the term *ethnographic perspective*, the aim would be to convey, in a relatively shorthand form, a sense of acceptance of a number of assumptions about research activity and the derivation of knowledge. These would include the use of naturalistic or fieldwork methods, interactionist approaches to analysis of data such as analytic induction or grounded theory, and an attempt to share in the social world or culture of the informants in order to elucidate the meaning of the actions themselves. It would also perhaps mean a perspective in which epistemological subtleties are seen to be less important than the pursuit of naturalistic data from the field. Both Hammersley and Atkinson (1983) and more recently Layder (1993) could be said to represent this tradition. The point about epistemological subtlety is not misplaced when the view of Anne Williams (1989) is considered. She amply illustrates the contextual nature of method and ethics whatever perspective is assumed in her description of the 'everyday messy life of the ethnographer' (p329).

Summary

I have provided an overview of the influences and specific perspective which have given me guidance in this work. To return briefly to the notion of epistemological pluralism, I would argue that many events in the natural sciences are amenable to investigation by means of rigorous measurement and the analysis of nominal data by means of the wide range of inferential statistics available. I would even accept that in the social and behavioural sciences, a good deal can be learned from the considered use of inferential statistics where concepts are well defined, samples are rigorously derived and of appropriate size.

I remain sceptical, however, that much that counts as quantitative nursing research meets these criteria and rather, statistics are used to add, just as with the third person singular style, a spurious objectivity to studies which attempt too often to quantify the unquantifiable. In these circumstances therefore, I have little confidence in epistemological pluralism if it renders studies incoherent as a result of the necessary reduction in size and energy used for either the qualitative or the quantitative analysis. As for this study, I claim to follow broadly a symbolic interactionist perspective. As may be evident, however, the influences of conflict positions and the social philosophy of Foucault (1991) have had an increasing part to play in my development over the course of this work.

2 Analytic approach

I have suggested that I will be working from a broadly symbolic interactionist perspective in the collection and interpretation of data. Within this tradition there remains a good deal of debate about the merits of various approaches to analysis and collection of data. An important point is that early anthropologists and ethnographers almost certainly gave little thought to such procedural matters. They made detailed notes of their observations, often in the form of a diary, and then wrote a description of events and phenomena as they saw things. Sometimes and where it was possible to do so, they would interview informants informally to check out their interpretation. The emphasis was on description of the social context they studied, and little or no claim was made to the generation or testing of formal theory. William Foote Whyte's (1955) *Street Corner Society* used this approach. Dingwall (1977) notes that accounts such as this were always open to the criticism, notably from positivistic social scientists, that such descriptions were 'mere journalism' and lacked credibility in any scientific sense.

Probably in order to defend qualitative research from such criticism, substantial energy was put by some workers into developing procedures for analysis (and collection) of data which would at least demonstrate how interpretations were derived. Probably because research reports were commonly being evaluated by the criteria accepted for scientific or positivistic research, attempts were often made to satisfy aspects of these criteria. Very large sample sizes were sometimes used even by noted Chicago School interactionists in an attempt to give the appearance of representativeness and therefore generalisability (e.g. Hughes', 1958 *Twenty Thousand Nurses Tell Their Story*).

A number of systematic approaches developed, of which analytic induction and grounded theory are perhaps the best known examples. Znaniecki (1934) proposed the use of a hypothetico-deductive model for the analysis of data and the testing of hypotheses in qualitative research. This approach, called analytic induction, can be briefly described as follows. The researcher identifies a rough definition of the problem to be studied. A hypothesis (or a statement of a relationship between variables) is formulated and a single case study is then examined to verify or refute the hypothesis. If the hypothesis is supported then more cases are collected and analysed in relation to it. A single negative case causes either refutation of the theory or a reformulation of the statement of the theory in terms of its hypotheses. Hammersley (1992) argues that whilst analytic induction is often appealed to by ethnographers as a model for their analysis, there are very few examples of its full and explicit implementation. He goes on to suggest furthermore that the large number of cases needed and the preponderance toward interviews only are discrepant with most ethnographic studies.

Grounded theory

First described fully by Glaser and Strauss (1967) in their book *The Discovery of Grounded Theory*, this approach has been used by an increasing number of researchers who utilise a sociological perspective, most particularly in the education (Meighan, 1986) and health fields (Morse and Johnson, 1991). Despite this trend, it is clear that exactly how to use the ideas and procedures involved has been a matter of either a great deal of interpretation or even misunderstanding. Strauss, in his more recent publication with Juliet Corbin (1990), admits that some of the responsibility for this lay with the original book, which is rather abstract and uses the first chapters to attack structural functionalist verificationism. Perhaps as a strategy for dealing with the ambiguities in the 1967 statement, some researchers have argued that their own approach takes a modified grounded theory approach (Kratz, 1974; Melia, 1987; Smith, 1992).

Whilst such honesty is creditable, it seems to me now, having worked with the approach directly, that modifications are not only defensible, they are inevitable. This inevitability almost obviates the need for the term modified. Such strategies as are adopted under the contingencies of the research setting and in analysis, provided they are made explicit, should be seen not as modifications but as legitimate flexibility and as developments of the original approach.

In recent years a number of systematic summaries and expositions of the analytic procedures of grounded theory have come to be available to the specialist and to the more general research student alike. Whilst (sadly) widely read research reports in book form commonly have the barest of one-page descriptions of the method (e.g. Smith, 1992) this is understandable from some publishers' point of view. Original theses such as Kappeli (1984), however, have a very clear account and are worth pursuing by postgraduates. Stern (1985) and Morse and Johnson (1991) give suitable outlines for the novice along with examples. By far the most detailed account of the procedures of grounded theory is to be found in the authoritative text by Strauss and Corbin (1990). Taking a practical and very well documented approach, this book contains the whole recipe with other guidance for researchers on topics such as writing reports and presenting papers. Their disclaimer that the book is meant for beginners rather than advanced students probably relates to the absence of much discussion of questions of epistemology or of the criticisms of various kinds which the approach has received. Nevertheless I have found the text extremely useful as a source of ideas, especially when confronted by analytic blockages.

Constant comparative analysis

In the *Discovery of Grounded Theory* Glaser and Strauss (1967) suggest that, as they use the term, constant comparative analysis can be applied to any level of organisation. They seem to suggest that qualitative analysis proceeds by comparing groups or individuals in order to make general statements about similarities and differences. Later work by Strauss and Corbin (1990), reduces this emphasis and suggests that comparisons are mostly of a conceptual nature. That is, instances of phenomena, once identified, are compared and contrasted in various ways and along different dimensions. Nevertheless the term *constant* gives the flavour of their intention. Analysis and collection of data are meant to proceed simultaneously, so that issues which arise out of, say, early observational notes may guide the further collection of data. The strategic rather than probabilistic identification of informants or other data sources has been called *theoretical sampling.*

Theoretical sampling

Strauss and Corbin (1990:176) define theoretical sampling as: "..sampling on the basis of concepts that have proven theoretical relevance to the evolving theory". Their choice of 'proven' is I suggest in its lay sense of 'shown', since formal proof is not a serious concern of the grounded theorist at any stage. This could happen when concepts repeatedly occur (or not) as incidents are compared. Therefore theoretical sampling might guide the selection of informants who are judged to be able to shed light upon an emerging theme. As I suggest later, the theme of unpopularity emerged early on in the collection of my data, so that as I proceeded I began to focus more upon this both in formal interviews and in my observations in Howarth ward.

Theoretical samples are seen to be appropriate when developing rather than testing theory, in which latter case strategies for randomisation become more important. The random sampling approach is necessary when some claim to statistical representativeness of wider populations is to be made, in which case the necessary sample size and appropriate inferential statistics are also required. Random samples should, however, play no part in grounded theorising. Indeed, when dealing with small numbers of respondents randomisation can lead to samples which are less rather than more representative.

Recording of data

In a sense, the recording of data is itself an aspect of the analysis. Inevitably choices are made about which data to observe, and which to remember, and then which to write down, and in what way. Both the books by Bogdan and Taylor (1975) and Schatzman and Strauss (1973) give guidance which is helpful. I decided to keep a pocket notebook, which was common practice among the nursing staff, in which I noted key phrases in ward (change of shift) reports. Occasionally I would retreat to the sluice, bathroom or kitchen to make some notes, but found that what Dingwall (1977) describes as "ethnographer's bladder" (frequent trips to the toilet to make notes) was unnecessary. However I was not operating covertly and so I could openly write in my book from time to time as did my colleagues. I learned a salutary lesson, however, when early in my data collection I mislaid the book which, at that time, had quite sensitive patient-related information in it. This situation caused me a good deal of grief and taught me that assurances about confidentiality depend not just on integrity but rigid security of notebooks and other raw data. Fortunately I retrieved the book in the hospital shop the day after with some confidence that it had been secure. It could have been otherwise and I still feel guilty about the possible hurt this data insecurity could have caused.

I also kept a small portable (pocket type) tape recorder, but I used this only for formally arranged interviews (with informants' consent) and to make quick summaries of my day's activities in the car on the way home.

Later that day I would transfer my fieldnotes from both formats to A4 sheets with dates, times, staff on duty and shift pattern. I used four main headings for these types of notes. *Empirical* meant those notes relating to what I had seen or heard and what I had been doing as a nurse participant on the ward. *Method* was a set of notes where I recorded technical issues as they arose. *Personal* was a set of notes about my feelings and personal experiences. As other ethnographers have found (Hammersley and Atkinson 1983), the personal and method aspects of a study can dominate a report. Whilst important in order to write reflexively, they should be held in the proper perspective in the final report. Finally at this stage it is important to make theoretical notes (or memos), which will help in further analysis. These consist of occasional flashes of inspiration, but more commonly a diligent recording of ideas from other studies or from other contexts which may have a bearing upon the analysis. Each day of my fieldwork I made sure I completed these tasks before doing anything else. Often the distinction between classes of notes so blurred that all were contained in the same stream of notes, a pattern which dominated my later data collection. The same became true of my transcripts when, after a few days, I began to do formally arranged interviews with my co-participants in Howarth Ward. Regularly every few days, however, I was able to read through both interview and field notes and re-classify the issues into these four main domains at the stage of open coding.

Open coding

Open coding is a process of reading through fieldnotes, interviews and even sometimes relevant literature, to identify issues, concepts or themes. The level of detail employed is largely personal choice. I wished to analyse every section of data for its meaning in the context in which it occurred. A section of data would commonly be a sentence or paragraph. I would then attach a label in the margin, usually a short phrase or word which had commonly but not exclusively a process orientation. Examples were 'toeing the line', and in the case of my personal notes, 'feeling the pressure'. Once I had done this for all my notes, I listed the labels on large A3 sheets of card in columns. In each case the label was identifiable by a date, page number and respondent code where appropriate. The simple expedient of coloured highlighter pens then helped me group labels under main category headings.

Having done this, and through repeated reading of the notes and labels, groups of labels which seem to fit in relation to one another are noted. It is important to be very diligent about identification of page numbers, sources of labels (such as respondent numbers) and dates. This is so that cross reference can easily be made when, with the passage of time, the origins of labels come to be engulfed by the vast amounts of data generated. The grouping of the labels and the data chunks, or as Melia (1981) describes them 'packages' is an important first stage in the analysis but one beyond which some researchers do not seem to progress.

The study by Stockwell (1972), which was probably the first British study by a nurse to attempt grounded theory, is an example of a study claiming to utilise grounded theory but where the report contains no evidence of attempts to analyse qualitative data systematically in order to discover categories and the hypothesised relations between them. Indeed as Hammersley (1992) suggests, progress beyond this first descriptive phase to a 'theory' may be less legitimate than Strauss and his various co-workers would claim.

It seems to me, though, that much of the debate about the theoretical status of grounded theory rests upon definitions of theory. With a typically broad view, Strauss and Corbin (1990) are happy to see this first level as what Stevens (1979) calls descriptive theory. Later stages of theory development would include elements of explanation, at which point the theory is labelled *substantive* in relation to its context of derivation. After much further work and in some cases incorporating predictive elements, the theory becomes, in Straussian terms *formal theory.*

Axial coding and the 'paradigm model'

Axial coding follows open coding is:

> A set of procedures whereby data are put back together in new ways after open coding, by making connections between categories. This is done by utilising a coding paradigm involving conditions, context, action/interactional strategies and consequences. (Strauss and Corbin, 1990:96)

Strauss and Corbin have been most helpful in their recent publication by outlining of this aspect of grounded theorising. When confronted by a mass of notes and basic concepts drawn from the written data-base, the task of making some kind of intelligent (and believable) inferences is awesome. To help the investigator to begin to make some sense of the data, Strauss and Corbin propose a paradigm or framework through which to view the data as a whole and the concepts as they emerge. This paradigm model, despite its title, is a straightforward framework with which to analyse concepts. As concepts enlarge (that is many concepts are organised around the one which seems to cover them all) it is helpful to think about them in process terms. Describing the phenomenon in question, such as 'brilliant nursing', it makes sense to describe the contexts in which it occurs, and the strategies that nurses adopt in order to carry it out. It is helpful to explain what is meant by the term, that is the meanings that nurses (and others) seem to attach to the term. Finally it is relevant to attempt to elucidate the consequences of 'brilliant nursing'. Some of these may be for the nurse, such as being seen to be deviant, or on a more positive note, job satisfaction. Other outcomes would be for the client.

This is the initial relevance of the Strauss and Corbin (1990) paradigm model. As a broadly process-oriented framework, it provides the basis for wider discussions of categories or even for chapters dealing with categories or themes arising from the data. However, I would stress that to be confined by the model described in the textbook would be limiting. In any work at all by Strauss and his colleagues, of which a very great deal is available, their flexibility in using the model merely as a guide is very evident. Sometimes in the research report for example, the consequences are less detailed than, say, the context. A further point is that, being rather procedurally detailed, strict allegiance to the letter of the Strauss and Corbin (1990) text would limit the very creativity which they themselves wish to encourage.

Selective coding

Strauss and Corbin (1990) strongly suggest that to have a number of categories in which data can be described and explained is very well, but that every effort should be made to organise the report under one single overarching category. This is termed selective coding and in my case this would be *social judgement.* In large works this may not be possible, but the effort involved in searching for conceptual links between data sections is rewarding, despite the demands it makes.

In both axial coding and selective coding I made a good deal of use of 8" by 5" cards upon which my data chunks (suitably cross-referenced) were written. Photocopies of original data sheets can be used, cut and pasted, but I found that hand-writing the data caused me to become immersed in the issues in a way which I should have found difficult with too many short-cuts.

Recent developments in computer data-base software such as *Nudist* have potential to sort through data very quickly for particular phrases or conceptual labels. However, in terms of visual presentation there is still much to be gained from spreading all the cards on the floor and letting human intuition play a part in the analysis. Computers with large screens, large memories and multi-window facilities could possibly assist in these tasks. I think that computers should increasingly play a part in qualitative analysis, provided that the computer technology does not cause a reversion to counting concepts rather than thinking about them. Coding procedures are concurrent and ought to be seen as flexible. They provide a framework and a method through which to begin to collect and to organise data in grounded theory, and which assist in producing a focus on process or interactional elements of the situation under study.

Some weaknesses of grounded theory

In perhaps the most widely quoted critique, George Brown (1973) attacks grounded theory from a positivist perspective, arguing that theory development ought not to be restricted to what appears relevant to research subjects. He suggests that only a certain type of data seems to be relevant to grounded theorists, and criticises their confidence in data which, for him, would produce only hunches. He gives the example of spending time in the hospital where he did his work investigating social factors which relate to mental illness. He suggests that if a process of theorising was possible at all it would be too long drawn out. Brown makes a number of points about developing a theory of causation, for which as one might expect he would see quantitative studies as more valid and of greater reliability. He does, however, concede a place for original modes of developing early theory, from whence it might be refined and tested by more 'scientific' methods.

As if to respond to criticisms of the positivist variety, some qualitative researchers such as Stern (1985) suggest that the canons of reliability and validity can be applied to grounded theory, but in a different way. Stern, for example argues that reliability, whilst impossible in practice in the sense of repeatability, can be attained by checking research outcomes with respondents. This trend continues with the recent Strauss and Corbin (1990) book where they argue that grounded theory is a scientific method. They suggest that criteria of verification and generalisability, for example, can be met. All that is required is re-definition of the terms.

I would suggest, in common with Hammersley (1992), that to deny a completely different epistemology is not an effective strategy. To meet criteria by redefinition of accepted scientific terms seems rather less intellectually satisfying than justifying the importance of new canons. Hammersley and Atkinson have done as much as anyone to generate appropriate canons or criteria of evaluation of ethnographic research (including grounded theory) such as reflexivity and relevance.

Hammersley (1992) does continue to utilise the concept of validity as a criterion for the assessment of ethnographic texts, but he seems to suggest that this assessment is a judgement made by the reader. He argues that validity depends upon the research being *credible* and *plausible*. Together with *relevance* and *importance* Hammersley concludes that studies should be seen to have contributed to available knowledge and understanding.

Barney Glaser (1992), one of the original authors of the grounded theory approach has criticised the Strauss and Corbin (1990) approach as excessively rigid and procedural. Indeed the critique is highly personalised giving the impression of a serious rift between Glaser and Strauss on more than theoretical differences. In one sense, Glaser's points make some sense, since the 1990 Strauss and Corbin approach has a definite flavour of the verificationism that the 1967 book attacked so vigorously.

It might reasonably be argued that any attempt to describe the social world with the accuracy implied by the rigid and doctrinal procedures in the later book, would be just as much a positivistic enterprise as any quantified approach. It would make assumptions about the permanence of concepts and the degree to which individuals would agree on their definition which are much more the province of the positivist than the phenomenologist or symbolic interactionist. I share some of these concerns, especially when, as nurses, we have something of a reputation for writing and adhering to procedures rather than being imaginative and creative in our work. With this in mind, one might hazard a guess as to the influence of Juliet Corbin (the nurse) in the detailed proceduralisation of the grounded theory approach in the 1990 book.

Summary of analytic procedures

I have attempted to give an overview of my use of the grounded theory method developed and outlined by Glaser and Strauss (1967) and later by Strauss and Corbin (1990). It seems to me that, though perhaps seeming over-structured at first, the method can still allow a good deal of creativity and flexibility of interpretation. The coding procedures and the paradigm model are helpful in the way that logical guides and procedures are helpful in gaining confidence with any skill, such as teaching. My experience of supervision of small scale qualitative research in my role as a teacher leads me to believe that students achieve deeper levels of analysis and synthesis of ideas about their data through the flexible use of such guides.

The analytic devices suggested by these writers also help to break the situation described by Stern (1985) and which most researchers recognise:

> The process may sound as if it occurs in a series of orderly steps, but it does not. The researcher may have dry spells (limited ideas) and may feel depressed. It seems that the deepest feelings of depression come before a creative breakthrough of ideas, or when the researcher feels most confused and begins to write. A high optimistic mood often occurs when the ideas come together and take form. (Stern, 1985:158)

This having been said it will be important in future work to expand the definition of grounded theory in the way suggested by Derek Layder (1993). He argues that some of the more powerful criticisms of this analytic approach arise out of the perhaps too-systematic application of the procedures so elaborately explained in books like Strauss and Corbin

(1990). Stern is right, that flexibility and some freedom is necessary if theory development is to be insightful and creative. Rigidity is not rigour!.

3 Participant observation

Fieldwork and participant observation

The research approach I take in this study grew out of my increasing belief that qualitative methods are the best approach when the substantive research area and its concepts are unclear and insufficiently developed. Previously I had used the survey approach with a Likert scale to attempt to examine student nurses' moral and other values (Johnson, 1983). The experience was most valuable, but it became clear that to use conceptual categories developed *a priori* and outside the context of the nurses' work was inappropriate. The analysis of the cross-sectional quantitative data showed some interesting and statistically significant findings, one of which was that the third year students valued altruism rather less than first years.

It was, however, frustrating to have little insight into the experiences the students were having which may have led to these results. A further consideration was my increasing interest in, and affiliation to, interpretive or broadly humanistic approaches to research. Here I intend to examine the method of participant observation in some detail, and within this review will be a consideration of interviewing. Schatzman and Strauss (1973) and others see this as part and parcel of participant observation, fieldwork or naturalistic sociology approaches.

Observer roles

In his much cited paper, Gold (1958) typifies four roles which an observer of a social setting may assume in order to collect data. In the role of complete observer, the researcher takes no deliberate part in events as they unfold and tries to record social phenomena as objectively as possible. Ashworth (1980) used this approach to collect data about the amount of communication which nurses engaged in with their highly dependent patients in intensive care units. She sat, for the main part of the study, on a chair placed in the corner of the unit clinical area where the nurses could be seen working closely with their patients and she recorded data using a checklist. I know how this felt, because I was one of the nurses she observed, and remember well my concern to clean my patient's mouth and eyes regularly when in fact Ashworth was studying our abilities to communicate verbally and non verbally with our unconscious charges! Popular among early and to some extent influential British nurse researchers such as Lelean (1973), Hawthorne (1974) and Bendall (1975), the complete observer method carries assumptions of objectivity and the passive role of the value-free scientist which are now more open to question. Schatzman and Strauss (1973) argue that whilst a researcher is visible to the hosts it is impossible for the researcher to have no effect on their behaviour. Indeed they stress that just by trying to look dispassionate and unaffected by what they see, complete observers will inevitably make informants nervous and cause them to behave differently:

> ...the spectre of a relatively impassive observer whether or not taking notes,... can be very disturbing to the hosts. (Schatzman and Strauss, 1973:59)

In this work, they suggest that the complete observer role, or what they term watching from outside, is virtually impossible to manage in natural settings and without technical assistance such as one-way mirrors. This said, technological developments in video cameras and radio microphones seem to be being tested by some researchers with the goal of unobtrusive data collection (Fielding, 1986; Rundell, 1991). Without such assistance, the terms used by Schatzman and Strauss (1973) namely 'passive presence' and 'limited interaction', give a false impression of the intention of the observer in this role.

Gold (1958) argues that next along the continuum of observer roles is 'observer as participant'. Here the investigator accepts a limited impact on the research setting and may, for example in action research, have a defined role in interacting with the hosts toward a specific aim whilst also collecting data. The model seems to fit the position taken in classic studies of medical student and nursing student socialisation such as those by Becker et al (1961) and Olesen and Whittaker (1967). These workers generally tried to follow their informants through as many of their day to day experiences as possible, but were also unlikely to participate in the specific work activities of their hosts, such as treatments and nursing care. Clearly the division is one of degree, since at a coffee break it was possible to be a more fulsome participant in that social activity than, say, personal nursing care. This was perhaps the more so because in most cases the researchers were sociologists and not members of the occupation being studied. The fluidity between some of these roles in practice is evident in the apparent differences of definition between commentators upon the roles. The influential Schatzman and Strauss (1973) seem to suggest that in the 'observer as participant' role the investigator participates more in events than Gold implies. They argue that this role is more suited to professionals doing research into their own discipline, and give the example of:

> ...a nurse, also trained as a sociologist, who works on a hospital ward whilst openly gathering data about features of life and interaction. (Schatzman and Strauss, 1973:61)

Given this lack of clarity, Gold (1958) calls this more involved participant role that of "participant as observer", putting the emphasis upon the participation. Despite their different terminology, Schatzman and Strauss (1973) see the more participative research role as less frequently attempted. This suggestion remains valid despite the fact that a limited number of nurses have attempted applied research into their own discipline and relatively few studies have appeared in the wider literature. Baker's (1978) study of routines of care in wards for the elderly exemplifies the approach, in that she undertook basic nursing duties whilst collecting her data so that she would experience the social world of her informants at first hand. Kappeli (1984) similarly worked closely with her nurse hosts caring for the elderly persons upon whom her study was focused. James (1986) worked as a staff nurse in a continuing care unit whilst she collected her data about the experience of this kind of nursing. Although using terms differently to Gold, Schatzman and Strauss (1973) suggest that, in the more participative role, the researcher has more 'active control' of data collection. In each of these studies the researcher identity of the individual was known, as far as possible, to potential informants.

In Gold's (1958) final category of observer role, that of 'complete participant', the role of the investigator is not disclosed to informants. This approach has been popular in the various branches of social science because of its apparent minimisation of the risk of hosts changing their behaviour in response to scrutiny. In the widely influential study by Rosenhan (1973) he and his co-workers mimicked mental illnesses so that they would experience the treatment of such persons in American psychiatric units. The report of an investigation by Field (1989) contains a smaller study in which a post-graduate student (Knight) took a post as a nursing auxiliary in order to examine covertly the experiences of dying patients and their nurses. The role of complete participant or as Schatzman and Strauss (1973) more descriptively term it 'participation with hidden identity' is clearly available to researchers, and has been used very recently in the United Kingdom by Clark (1996a and b). Many commentators such as Olesen and Whittaker (1967) and Baker (1978) distance themselves from it in view of the inconsistency of the necessary deception with humanistic methods. I review the main moral questions confronting the different forms of participant observer (including Clark) in chapter five on ethical issues, and discuss the deception by Field and Knight (Field, 1989) in some depth elsewhere (Johnson 1992).

To summarise the roles that may be taken, it seems that a large degree of overlap does, and should, exist between observer roles. In the initial phases of fieldwork, it seems sensible that the observer participates less and spends more time orientating to the research setting, collecting structural data, identifying work routines and discussing their research role with potential informants. Later in the research, the role may change to include, for the nurse researcher, a significant involvement in clinical nursing activity. This will depend upon the focus of the study and the degree to which 'doing nursing' (to borrow a category from Melia, 1981) will be helpful both in terms of bargaining for data and understanding the social world of those present.

In my own field work, I assumed mainly the role of participant as observer, that is to say that for the most part I worked as a supernumerary staff nurse. I stress that my identity as a researcher was open however.

Table 1: Observer roles in research (after Gold, 1958)

COMPLETE OBSERVER
OBSERVER AS PARTICIPANT
PARTICIPANT AS OBSERVER
COMPLETE PARTICIPANT (COVERT)

Participant observation

The ensuing discussion aims to review the chief issues surrounding the method of participant observation. The term is seen by Ragucci (1972) as synonymous with ethnography because the method of participant observation is so commonly the mainstay of ethnography. Aamodt (1991:41) suggests that ethnography is a:

...way of collecting, describing, and analysing the ways in which human beings categorise the meaning of their world.

Ethnography is a term increasing in popularity under the influence of nurse anthropologists such as Leininger (1985) but the role of participant observation in gaining insights into systems and cultures is widely seen as fundamental. It is perhaps misleading to regard participant observation as a single method (McCall and Simmons, 1969). McCall and Simmons, whose edited collection of papers on the topic is a major resource, suggests the approach is a:

> ...characteristic blend of techniques, as exemplified by the work of the lone anthropologist living amongst an isolated people, (which) involves some amount of genuinely social interaction in the field with the subjects of the study, some direct observation of relevant events, some formal, and a great deal of informal interviewing, some systematic counting, some collection of documents and artefacts, and open endedness in the directions the study takes. (McCall and Simmons, 1969:1)

A very extensive literature on method is available to the student. Succinct histories of the intellectual and methodological origins of ethnography and participant observation are to be found in Bruyn (1966), McCall and Simmons (1969) and Dingwall (1977). A sociologist (Johnson, 1975) notes that the history of field research (participant observation) and ethnography is quite long and that the approaches were indeed drawn from early anthropological studies of 'primitive' communities. Later workers of the Chicago School popularised the approaches for the analysis of social life in Urban America. Generally speaking however those sociologists developing *Grand Theory* and using quantitative analysis of survey data were for a considerable period of time the most influential. This may have been, as Melia (1981) argues, because of the coincidental development of computers with the power to analyse data quickly as well as the fact that these methods were seen to mimic the more respectable physical sciences.

A number of studies using the participant approach continued to be published by a minority of enthusiasts such as Whyte (1955) and Becker et al (1961). Becker was developing a reputation for converting the interpretive or broadly symbolic interactionist perspective into qualitative data which could, with some effort, be analysed to bring forth alternative perceptions of the social world of those studied. These perceptions were seen as necessary because much work had previously tried to explain the roles and functions of individuals in terms of existing *armchair theory*. Becker's chief method was participant observation and he was able to show quite convincingly that his approach did seem to describe accurately

24

the students' experiences of occupational socialisation in a Kansas medical school.

Glaser and Strauss (1967), having worked with Becker and his colleagues, were similarly convinced of the need to see social reality in the terms and concepts of those experiencing the phenomena under study. Their work may have had wide appeal because it generally examined the sensitive if taboo subject of the experiences of the dying and those who care for them. Glaser and Strauss's ability to identify from their data concepts which, though new to the literature, were ones with which nurses and others could identify, may have enhanced their appeal. Concepts such as the social loss of dying patients (Glaser and Strauss, 1964), awareness of dying, and trajectories of dying had a descriptive and explanatory power which would inevitably convince some researchers that both perspective and method had much to offer.

This group of researchers remained small throughout the 1970s in the United States, the most significant work being done by nurses who were actually associates of Strauss and Glaser, such as Quint (1967). In the United Kingdom the participant observation method was used by Dingwall (1977) in a major study of the social organisation of health visitor training. In the study he followed Becker's (1961) model of accompanying the students in as many of their professional and day to day social activities as possible. Kratz (1978) used participant observation to describe the care of the long-term sick, notably stroke patients, in the community. She draws explicitly upon the symbolic interactionist perspective and acknowledges the influence of Becker and Glaser and Strauss. Kratz freely discusses the problems, both sociological and professional which using the approach caused her in collecting her data. As a sociologist she felt that she had only to co-operate in care at a basic level and to record what she saw and heard. As a nurse, dealing often with persons in dire need of improved resources and better standards of care, she felt very much the need to intervene on moral grounds. The chain of influence from the early days in Chicago, was clearly extending through Dingwall and now Kratz, to a small number of nurse researchers such as Dorothy Baker (1978). Baker undertook an ambitious study of the care of the elderly in different wards and under the direction of ward sisters with different styles of management of care.

She too acknowledges the debt to Strauss and Glaser more in terms of her method than in terms of her analytic procedures, and seems also to have influenced workers in this field such as Reed and Bond (1991). At this point, however, some sympathisers with the symbolic interactionist perspective seem to begin to reduce the importance of true participant observation and argue instead that interviews with respondents are as useful in generating accounts of phenomena in the terms of those involved. Two students of both Kratz and Baker have provided important insights into the student nurse's social world, but using no observational procedures as most understand them. Melia's (1981,1987) widely referred to accounts of student nurses' work and training used only interviews with the respondents, as did Luker's (1984) analysis of the nurse undergraduates' management of their perceived 'differentness' from traditional (RGN) nursing students.

Melia (1981), in her Ph.D. thesis argues that what she calls the 'informal interview' is virtually a form of participant observation, and that data though not the same are 'not greatly different'. It is perhaps worth exploring briefly here Melia's (1981) suggestion that her method of interviewing respondents was 'informal' (p.48). She scheduled appointments with her student informants and did some of the interviewing in her own flat and taped the conversations. This might seem to be informal in that she had only a loose agenda of issues on a card, and took an admittedly 'conversational' approach. Melia draws very heavily for her justification of method upon Schatzman and Strauss's (1973) *Field Research: Strategies for a Natural Sociology*. On this issue however, they see her approach as quite 'formal' because it was planned and systematic. Melia seems to draw her concept of informality from the conversational nature of the meeting, but this is perhaps better defined as semi- or loosely structured.

The point may seem small, but it suggests that through the use of ethnographic language Melia (1981) is making a case that her method was closer to the field or the work setting of the students than is really so. Whilst acknowledging that participant observation is almost synonymous with qualitative method and that 'participant observation stresses the part played by the researcher in the generation of data' (p.47) Melia (1981) goes on to justify her decision to use only formal interviews (to use the Straussian definition and not her own). She does this by arguing that:

...the distinction between interview and participant observation...is not such a clear cut one when data collection and analysis are considered empirically rather than conceptually. (Melia, 1981:48)

Pam Smith (1992) defends Melia's conception of interviewing as participant observation in both Melia's case and for that part of her own study which relied mostly upon interviews. I have discussed many of these points with Kath Melia (personal communication, 1996) and I believe that her interviews were conducted with a strong sense of integrity to the fieldwork and in the feeling that students were indeed conveying the 'essence' of their experiences. I also recognise that I have focused on Kath Melia's example alone when in fact there has grown up a whole tradition of research conducted by means of the 'ethnographic interview'.

Where Melia and I differ, I think, is in the degree to which other researchers influenced by Melia's evident success with this approach, are likely to conduct their 'ethnographies' by interview alone because it is easier to negotiate access, quicker, more practical and avoids some of the ethical and emotional difficulties.

I maintain therefore, and with the wider nursing research scene in mind, that (true) participant observation is undertaken only with reluctance. This is despite Schatzman and Strauss's (1973) claim that it is the essence of qualitative research strategy, (i.e. essential). Within the qualitative tradition in nursing the method has certainly never become very popular in comparison with the semi-structured interview, and participant observation in true clinical settings such as in the study by James (1986) remains a relative rarity.

To summarise, whilst there is a long tradition of participant observation in sociology and anthropology, the method has met with only limited enthusiasm in health care research. Nurses in both America and Britain have been reluctant to use the approach despite the increasing claims to the importance of ethnographic and humanistic perspectives by nurse researchers such as Field and Morse (1985).

Advantages of participant observation

Schatzman and Strauss (1973:5) suggest that for the ...naturalistically oriented humanist the choice of method is virtually a logical imperative. By this they seem to mean that it is acceptable to be committed to a research method before the research problem is defined:

> Conventional wisdom suggests that a researcher prepare a relatively articulated problem in advance of the enquiry... Yet, the field method process of discovery may lead the researcher to (his) problem after it has led (him) through much of the substance in (his) field. (p3)

This view is at least an honest one, compared to the common assertion that researchers choose their method according to the nature of the problem to be investigated. It does seem that researchers are often trained in a particular approach and then investigate suitable problems rather than the other way round. Despite the personal and almost intuitive commitment that enthusiasts for participant observation feel, it is also rational and honest to identify the clear practical and theoretical advantages to the approach before attempting it to examine a particular substantive research area.

Since my research area is broadly the subjective experience of confronting moral problems in nursing, I have attempted to show some of the theoretical advantages to participant observation in relation to the

27

investigation of this area (Johnson, 1990). In the paper I argue that there are perhaps three ways in which the moral values and knowledge base of nursing have been derived. These approaches can be loosely termed experience, deduction and empiricism. The experiences of early nurses in controlling infection without an adequate knowledge of microbiology led to a predominance of rules and procedures upon which nurses organised their work. With its militaristic and religious background nursing also drew from rules, procedures and traditions for the moral values which underpinned practice. Commonly these values, learned through the process of occupational socialisation, included obedience to medical authority and 'fitting in' with local practices (Melia, 1987). In the 1960s and 70s British nursing came increasingly under the influence of American academic nurses who deductively derived much of their 'theory' of nursing and how it ought to be practised from popular psychological, sociological and biological theories of the day. Clear examples of behaviourism, social systems and stress-adaptation theories are to be found in Orem (1980) and Roy (1980). The third method of generating nursing knowledge, empiricism, is based upon systematic analysis of nursing practice as it *is*, rather than as it *ought* to be as Orem, Roy and a number of others describe it. This approach is exemplified by the ethnographic and other qualitative approaches of Baker (1978), Smith (1992) and to some extent by Benner (1984).

This latter approach is, I argue, better suited to the study of moral questions in nursing than either drawing upon traditions or grand theories in isolation. I recognise that from a philosophical standpoint, purely empirical methods will not necessarily allow the production of improved moral positions or behaviour. However, I make the point that the case material usually used in the debate of moral questions is most frequently that produced either by the medical profession or the law. I therefore argue that there is a case for applied *naturalistic* sociology to enrich this debate with material which more nearly approximates the perspectives of the people involved such as patients and their carers. I argue that grounded theory could be well suited to this role, providing new insights into the values and the questions seen to be important by those experiencing health care most directly. In conclusion I suggest that it would then be fruitful to use moral perspectives such as utilitarianism and human rights to evaluate practices from a moral standpoint.

Gans (1968) focuses his discussion of the advantages of participant observation upon the central idea that the researcher is the instrument of data collection and analysis of data. This he argues puts the researcher "close to the data", a point amplified by Bailey (1985) who suggests that the method not only allows first hand witnessing of events, but allows the hosts to display "ordinary behaviour". This is clearly in contradistinction to the quasi-experimental methods of many social psychologists who have drawn far-reaching conclusions about human behaviour from artificially constructed experimental conditions such as the supposed electrocution of persons in a 'learning' experiment (Milgram, 1963). The idea that hosts will display ordinary behaviour is disputed by Knight and Field (Field, 1989), who felt that they had to use covert methods to study the nursing of dying patients in one surgical ward. They claim that the covert observation undertaken by Knight was done so that "communication and general behaviour were natural and normal" (p.35) which suggests a lack of faith in the value of data obtained by open means. Paradoxically Field's main study (1989) uses primarily the semi-structured interview method in which his identity and broad research agenda were clearly known to respondents. Most advocates of participant observation suggest that if participants' behaviour does alter, then this is only in limited ways and for a limited period, since the strategy for access and becoming accepted is designed to engage the trust of the hosts (Schatzman and Strauss, 1973).

Given that the researcher's identity is known to the hosts, then Colledge (1979) proposes that the approach minimises the need for role pretence. In his paper, which perhaps attempts to address many complex issues in little space, Colledge nevertheless summarises a number of benefits of the participant observer approach. Citing Leininger (1970) he suggests that the method should give:

> ...an accurate and fairly reliable picture of the cultural group or a patient's cognitions of health and illness. (p142)

This perhaps rather optimistic aim uses the concept of reliability in its lay sense rather than its technical one, since the method applied in other settings must necessarily discover different data (and is therefore unreliable in the technical sense of unrepeatable). It conveys the intent of describing and explaining the social world of those observed in their own terms, however. Stern (1985) addresses the reliability issue by stressing that replication is impossible, and that reliability is established by asking respondents to evaluate findings. Here too the concept of reliability is stretched to mean something more akin to validity, that is that the data record what is actually happening rather than that they are repeatable in other settings.

To summarise, there are technical advantages to the method of participant observation which include being very close to the data, being able to follow up leads and hunches, being able to validate emerging theory continuously in the context in which it is most relevant, and to experience the social world of informants in a way that the interviewer in an office or other setting cannot. The theoretical advantages include the opportunity to construct an account of phenomena in the terms of the persons involved directly, rather than in those of researchers' journal articles or case reports.

Problems with participant observation

In his very open and substantial treatment of the subject of participant observation Dingwall (1977) classifies the problems which relate to the method as scientific, political and ethical. These broad categories seem useful if it is acknowledged that they overlap a good deal and that some issues appear under all headings. In the following discussion I will address principally the first two categories, leaving discussion of the main ethical issues I confronted to a separate section.

'Scientific' problems

In his defence of the approach, Dingwall (1977) notes that participant observation has been attacked as 'mere journalism'. This is perhaps because there is considerable room for observer bias in reporting phenomena. Researchers are often keen to demonstrate their pet 'hobby horse', and this may be evident. However, eminent quantitative social and behavioural scientists such as Cyril Burt were also capable of misrepresenting research data to achieve their goals (Eysenck and Kamin, 1981). Whilst ethnographers may claim to be more honest about their bias (or perspective) this does not remove it. In the Glaser and Strauss (1967) grounded theory approach the concept of theoretical sensitivity is used to explain the researcher's pre-conceived notions of what may be important issues for study. These workers freely admit that they did not come upon their principal research interests by entering the field and then discovering that the care of dying persons was fraught with lies, deception and *closed awareness*. They had a good idea already from personal family experiences of their own . They were, as they put it, 'theoretically sensitive' from personal experience outside the research context.

This admission and the concept of theoretical sensitivity move some way to meet the problem of what to observe. The noted philosopher of science Karl Popper used to illustrate what is sometimes termed the *problem of induction* by asking his students to enter a room and 'observe'. They would commonly return, to Popper's satisfaction, asking *what* they should observe.

Popper's (1968) point is that it is impossible to collect data without at least some frame of reference or questions in mind, a view which differs from the grounded theory position only, it seems, in the degree to which the question or hypothesis has clarity and is defined in strict operational terms. In a more pragmatic discussion of this issue, Kappeli (1984) whilst owing allegiance to the open agenda approach of grounded theory in her observations, still notes the difficulty of deciding how to observe efficiently and not to miss instances of useful data. Fox (1982) argues that this very problem will lead inevitably to researchers collecting only those instances of data which support their desired research outcomes, much as politicians use only those examples which support their position. This, he argues seems less likely to be the case in complete observer studies such as those of Lelean (1973) or Ashworth (1980) where there were boxes to tick and columns to fill.

Another problem is the effect the observer has on the setting. It seems clear that in many situations, both journalistic and scientific, this effect declines in magnitude with increasing trust, acceptance and unobtrusiveness of the researcher with an adequately negotiated position. A great number of studies have revealed aspects of behaviour which at first sight it seems the hosts would have naturally wanted to conceal (Bell and Encel, 1978; Bulmer, 1982). It seems, however, that adequate guarantees of anonymity and confidentiality are helpful. Clearly television journalists find it so much more difficult to give such guarantees, and distort the images and voices usually only to protect those at personal risk of reprisals or criminal liability. It is interesting that in the different areas of social investigation, that is journalism and social research, principles of anonymity and confidentiality are so differently perceived.

Researcher or so-called *Hawthorne effect* is therefore not a fear for the participant observer. It is accepted that the social world described through the research activity is a construction of those involved, including the observer. Deliberate intervention is openly discussed, as an aspect of researcher *reflexivity*, and the report of the research is intended to be read with this in mind.

Faugier (1981) draws attention to the exhausting nature of participant observation. She studied an alcoholic treatment unit using the method and had to give due consideration to concentration span when trying to seem unobtrusive and yet observe and record significant events. Baker (1978) and Kappeli (1984) worked in elderly care wards where typically resources are minimal and the need for hard physical work to maintain even minimal acceptable standards of nursing was very evident. As part of the 'bargain' for data, being helpful and doing a fair share of physical work is tempting. It seems important to be realistic and, as Schatzman and Strauss (1973) suggest, if participation is too demanding of energy and time then research suffers.'Going native' has long been recognised as a problem in anthropological research, and the particular moral pressures which a nurse may feel in a very busy environment to work rather than watch must be a great inducement to see research activity as of lower priority.

31

I found that starting a shift at the same time as my co-participants demonstrated my willingness to be there when the work was allocated (so that I got my fair share). Where I worked an early shift (7.30 start) this meant that I could leave early at lunch time to engage in my writing up and this was understood to be reasonable. Even so, I soon became drained of energy with the constant awareness of wishing to use the time effectively to collect data and yet remain more useful to my colleagues than a complete observer.

Political problems

Punch (1986) gives a vivid account of the difficulties which may be experienced when doing fieldwork in an organisational setting. Dingwall (1977) also seems keen to suggest that observation fits poorly into settings with a hierarchical administration and the development of sets of routine management procedures. He seems to be saying that the method ought not to be a means of collection of information for managers, and that a good deal of distance ought to exist between researcher and managers, so that the investigator is not seen by participants in the study as a 'spy'. Baker (1978) went to some lengths after negotiating access with managers to distance herself from them. She avoided them and refused invitations to meet them in their offices as this might have been seen by her informants as evidence of her spy status. Despite knowing some of the senior staff I found it easy to avoid contacts with them and I am grateful to them for their tact in this respect.

Dingwall (1977) makes the valid point that participant observation is politically neutral but that the context in which it takes place is not. There is an inevitable conflict of interests between any number of competing groups in complex health care settings. More than ever, competition between units and groups is of a market nature as a result of Government initiatives such as *Working for Patients* (Department of Health, 1989). This means that information on standards, quality of the service or other market-sensitive indicators is likely to be sought by those with other than purely academic interest. Investigators need therefore to be aware of the sensitivity of their information and treat its dissemination with due caution.

Within the framework of political problems it seems sensible to discuss some of the various role conflicts which observers may experience though these are, as I have suggested, hardly limited to this category. Peggy Ann Field (1990) discusses the difficulties which nurses confront when observing their own setting. Some of these relate to the preceding discussion of feeling the need to do too much clinical work to help out. Another key problem is what might be termed the moral dissonance of observing and participating in care which is at variance with the observer's own professional standards. This creates a need to decide upon the level of observer intervention which will be appropriate within the context of the research. This issue will be explored further in the section dealing with specific ethical issues of the participant observer role. Being an 'insider' is seen to involve slightly different role ambiguities. As a patient and, it seems, a covert observer, Delamont (1987) discusses her wish that she had disclosed her researcher identity to her informants who were women undergoing various gynaecological operations. This was as much to feel that she was not deceiving them as to be able to ask more in depth questions. She did however feel that, whatever her perceived identity, she would fit uneasily with her informants in terms of a host of personal factors. She was 'different': she was not one of the 'suburban women' whom she sought to study. She had no children, no husband, no visitors (from choice) and was having an elective hysterectomy unlike her co-participants, most of whom had a 'disease'. In summary, she felt greatly the almost inevitable social distance between her and her informants. Baker (1978) similarly discusses the social distance she felt between herself and her host co-participants. Interestingly she notes that despite her own relatively working class background the hosts perceived her, with a Southern accent, as middle class and therefore different from themselves with their mainly Northern working class background. Baker, like Delamont, says that she struggled for coffee-time conversation since she did not share their interest in television (she did not have one), and also lived alone with no children, a main topic of off-stage conversation among the married female nursing auxiliaries.

This discussion of some of the issues which may cause role conflict leads to consideration of personal characteristics and the role they may play in the management of researcher and participant identity. Burgess (1982) notes a number of variables which could affect the negotiation of the researcher role. He includes age, gender, ethnic origin and experience as factors to bear in mind. Whilst it seems useful to have such factors in mind, it seems futile to produce exhaustive lists of factors which may limit identification with the participants. Indeed the early ethnographers were almost invariably at an immense social distance from those they undertook to try to understand. Frequently they needed to learn a very difficult language. The point seems to be to maintain an awareness of oneself in the setting and to use research tactics to attempt to see and understand the participants' perspectives, whilst declaring limits to this understanding which may be due to any obvious social distance.

Personal role conflict

In an elegant piece of self-disclosure and intellectual honesty consistent with his humanist and naturalistic participant observer position, Dingwall (1977) offers to 'the sociological community' the role ambiguity he experienced when he extended his researcher-informant relationship with one of his respondents (student health visitors) to one of greater personal intimacy. He himself uses the term 'affair', and whilst he informs us that they were later married he concedes that this is irrelevant to the discussion since this could have been otherwise. Dingwall seems to suggest that such developments might be an inevitable consequence of humanistic sociology where the boundaries between researcher and researched are increasingly blurred. However he also seems to fear that such a relationship could be seen as an abuse of power in a privileged relationship which may be likened to that between a doctor and a patient.

I have deliberately discussed this issue here rather than in my chapter on ethical aspects because I will argue that, whilst the incident would clearly present problems, it has no essentially ethical character. Dingwall was, it seems, openly researching the social world of the health visitor students who were his hosts. He had no formal authority over them, and his special relationship was with a mature adult. He presumably had, as we all arguably have, interacted as humans do in the complex way that contains in all interaction some sexual aspects. They both simply chose, freely and from alternative courses of action, to develop the relationship from one level which was perhaps not controversial, to another which Dingwall perceives was worthy of concern. Dingwall freely admits his anxieties and seems to feel greatest concern over the need he and the woman concerned felt to conceal the liaison until the research was completed.

Dingwall is wise and brave to offer the incident for the scrutiny of sociologists (and nurses) using these methods in applied discipline research. He is wise because in our culture sexual relations between colleagues commonly cause interpersonal difficulties. They may be impractical, painful and in the face of misunderstanding could cause serious problems in the collection of data. As to whether they are unethical, I suggest that the position adopted by Harris (1975) is useful. He argues that sex, whatever form it takes, can only be wrong where there is 'violation, exploitation, the infliction of harm, pain (or) suffering' (p191). Whether Dingwall behaved unethically rests not upon whether he had sex with a respondent but upon whether he exploited this partner in some way or harmed her. From the evidence available I would conclude that he did not. Dingwall is brave because others would not make the disclosure and yet honesty is perhaps the most humanistic feature of participant observation, and the one which defeats many of the scientific and methodological objections to it.

Other personal difficulties are encountered by participant observers to which a number of writers draw attention. Gans (1968) discusses the fear of rejection by the hosts in the middle of the project due perhaps to some tactless blunder by the researcher. Kappeli (1984) describes her fear of 'not doing things in the right order' and what she felt was the awful 'slowness' of her data collection. Strauss and Corbin (1990) are reassuring in many of these respects because they suggest that even experienced observers worry a good deal over such matters. They do not pretend it is easy, but they inspire confidence, paradoxically, by describing their mistakes and tactical blunders. They are able to dispel to some extent the myth of their infallibility as experts and write encouragingly about the problems faced in fieldwork.

Negotiation of role

The preceding remarks upon some of the problems faced by participant observers are not exhaustive. Some examples of problems emerging in my study will be discussed in the context of the fieldwork and analysis of data.

It is useful to review the literature on the method to become sensitised to some of these issues so that avoidable problems are indeed avoided. What emerges from this process seems to be a form of what Kramer (1974) describes as anticipatory socialisation. That is the sensitisation of the neophyte to possible problems so that the reality shock is not so great or so incomprehensible. Awareness of the likelihood of discomfort in the method is calculated to enable the researcher to tolerate these difficulties and to behave constructively in dealing with them. One strategy for this is to negotiate the participant observer role very carefully with all concerned. Quite apart from the centrality of the concept of negotiation in the writing of the influential Strauss and his colleagues, he and Schatzman (1973) note particularly the importance for fieldworkers of thinking clearly about the roles they will play in the field and their limits.

Bogdan and Taylor (1975) note the main points of this process. First, they suggest telling the truth to the hosts. They seem to imply that a slight economy of the truth is acceptable, saying that one need not explain substantive or theoretical interests in great detail. Clearly there has to be a limit to the extent of explanation which satisfies the need for informed consent, because they argue that it is counterproductive to use esoteric research terminology. It seems important to bear the hosts' background in mind and give a more comprehensive account to those who may benefit. The advice they give is to be "honest but vague" (p35). How this works in the field is a different matter, and I found that I never knowingly needed to be 'vague' about my aims. Compared to more structured studies with very specific questions to ask, my aims were already vague. As my interest in *unpopularity* became clearer, however, I was honest that this was becoming a substantive area of interest along with certain others.

Bogdan and Taylor (1975) discuss the *bargain* which ought to be struck with gatekeepers and hosts. They suggest that one aspect is non-disruption of the setting. Baker (1978) calls this *unobtrusiveness* and notes the right of informants to make known to the investigator if they have become a nuisance. Trustworthiness is part of the bargain and is made clear partly by the distancing behaviour from management and explicit statements about how reports and other data will be protected and presented only in suitable anonymous forms. Acceptability was important to Baker (1978) and Kappeli (1984), and is to some extent gained by social exchange. Baker did her share of what her respondents saw as hard menial work in order to become accepted and to overcome the social distance created by her different lifestyle and her perceived 'ex-ward sister' status. Kappeli undertook a number of social roles which increased her acceptability, such as being a confidante to some of the nurses and a 'wailing wall', that is someone who could be complained and moaned to without taking action. Such roles may help increase acceptability but are not without their own stresses, as Williams (1989) notes. It becomes difficult to differentiate between legitimate research data gleaned in the researcher role, and data obtained in some role as friend or confidante which, Williams argues, it is unfair to use, however well disguised in the report. Perhaps this is what really troubled Dingwall in his relationship with his co-participant.

Role negotiation is not, it seems, amenable to simple rules. The stance taken needs to be contextual. Much can be gained by continual discussion with experienced colleagues, peers, and in many settings the co-participants. It will be made easier in the case of applied health researchers such as nurses when a wider and more available British literature addresses some of these issues. Much of value lies in original theses which unfortunately, when published in book form, are often abridged to eliminate discussion of these matters in any depth, such as that by Smith (1992).

Conclusion

I have suggested that nurse researchers in general have found it convenient to avoid participant observation despite its virtual imperative status in the view of enthusiasts like Strauss and Schatzman (1973). Such a position may well be justifiable on resource or other technical grounds. Participant observation is certainly very expensive in terms of time. Other explanations seem to me more likely, and these might include, anxiety, loss of confidence in clinical skills and potential role conflict. These things considered, they are in essence the difficulties of clinical nursing, notably when contact with the setting is short or when roles are not clearly defined as, for example in the case of the nurse teacher or lecturer who visits the clinical area infrequently to teach clinical nursing (Jones, 1983).

It may seem pompous of me to imply criticism of this avoidance behaviour, but I too have been in his situation. As a nurse teacher I slid from regular weekly sessions of clinical nursing in two wards to virtually no clinical contact over a period of only a year or so. My teaching colleagues at the time were happy to reward my 'good sense' since they too had retreated to the relative safety of the classroom and even more, the committee room. In my discussion of my fieldwork I give examples of the strain of returning to the physically and emotionally demanding labour of nursing. Even without attempting to 'think sociologically' and record data, this is very hard.

Perhaps as a result of these possible discomforts, which most nurses recognise if they are honest, there seems to me to be an inexorable slide towards safe (or hygienic) research. By this I mean research which avoids these problems for the most part, and instead focuses on more accessible issues which do not require the researcher's presence in protracted interaction with respondents or in the clinical setting.

Despite this, onn returning to clinical work in the research context, provided the area is well chosen clinical skills return quickly. Remaining in one setting is helpful, since trying to appear credible when you do not know even the ward layout or where things are kept is very difficult. Most of all, knowing the patients well makes playing a credible role either as researcher or teacher possible, and this can only be achieved by working consistently in the same area. As a means to obtain a wealth of rich data which has relevance to the setting participant observation has potential which has not yet been fully explored. In combination with some form of action research, the method could offer a very great deal in the solution of clinical problems.

4 Access and ethics

Chicago School ethnographers have a tradition of making the setting of their research very explicit even to the point of naming the institution they studied (see Becker et al, 1963). However, I have no intention of making clear where I undertook the investigation because my access was granted on condition of anonymity both of the institution and individuals.

At first I intended to undertake my study in a location fairly near to where I live for reasons of convenience. I wanted access to an ordinary suburban district general hospital so that my observations, whilst not necessarily being generalisable, would nevertheless not be too atypical. I received informal permission from one of the senior nurses to do some preparatory work, which really only involved a few days' experience of a ward to practise my interview skills and to see how difficult it would be to work and to make observations. I saw this as an educational experience and no more. A week before I was due to arrive however, the same nurse telephoned me to say it was off. She said that things were getting hot managerially, and in the current climate they could not afford any public criticism. Of course I accepted this, but with great disappointment. A week later the situation became national news when one of the nursing staff complained about poor standards of care due to underfunding and staff shortages. I think I then knew why they were nervous of my study, although I was keen to give assurances about confidentiality.

Spencer (1982) gives a detailed account of the obstacles which may be encountered in gaining access to bureaucratic elites. He is describing his problems in attempting to study an American Military Academy, but many of his points remain valid for large and increasingly market sensitive institutions such as hospitals. He lists among his reasons why access is sometimes not given as threat to personal careers, problems of legitimacy of the researcher, threat to the institution's power and the problem of exchange. By this he means that both sides should feel that they have something to gain. On this occasion I failed to meet the last two criteria since I was not clear about any benefit which the hospital might gain, and the institution was already threatened by the widespread media criticism of its standards.

With some initial reluctance, therefore, I approached one of a number of teaching hospitals where I thought that the senior nursing staff would be initially sympathetic to my request for access. I thought this because I knew them quite well through professional connections. My reluctance grew out of a wish to avoid any kind of networking, although I now believe that my fears that I would be seen to be spying for management were groundless. As it was, the two managers that I approached had substantial knowledge of research and I did not doubt their integrity, so I knew that whilst facilitating my initial access they would not expect me to report back to them in any way after my preparatory work or later that year in my main study.

I submitted a research proposal to the hospital research ethics committee but they did not require me to attend. On this occasion also I emphasised the substantial reputations of my main academic supervisors which may have added to my legitimacy in Spencer's (1982) terms. The committee seemed to take the view that, since no invasive or treatment procedures were involved, and since I had given assurances about anonymity and confidentiality, they would only expect a brief report of my progress by letter.

Although pilot studies in such work are not strictly necessary, I did undertake a period of a few days' observation in a ward where a large number of patients had a form of cancer, and learned, in particular, that I would need to adopt a role similar to that of bank staff nurse. This would allow me to help with the work using those skills which I still seemed to have (to a greater or lesser degree), as a means of gaining trust and acceptance, whilst avoiding full responsibility for planning and delivering nursing care.

The Director of Nursing suggested various wards to me, mostly based upon the criterion of the staff not being threatened, or being prepared to give it a try. My criterion was primarily that the ward should not be too specialised. I wanted to get some kind of insight into what Dingwall (1980:874) suggests is the commonplace routine rather than the good story. In terms of my interest in moral questions at the time, I also wanted to examine day to day issues rather than the big dilemmas (Thompson, Melia and Boyd, 1988).

I decided to approach the sister in charge of a general medical ward. I first wrote to her so that she could put the idea to her colleagues, and then went along to discuss it. Explaining in advance was quite difficult, but I tried to be honest about my background and my aims. In particular I said that whilst I did not wish to be on the off duty so that I would remain supernumerary, I was prepared to work on each shift in the ordinary way. We agreed the date that I would start, and I stressed that I would be there at the standard time of 7.30 a.m.. I would probably work from four to five shifts per week, but these would commonly be until lunch time. I worked a slightly smaller number of shifts in the afternoons, and these were usually fruitful opportunities for dialogue with both patients and staff. Occasionally I would work a different shift, such as from 4 p.m. to 9-30 p.m., and I worked until 2 a.m. twice to meet night staff.

The ward

The ward was an upgraded Nightingale type with three bays for six patients each, and three side wards on the corridor near to the ward office, treatment room and kitchen. On this corridor lay also a doctors' office, and a linen cupboard and store room. Thus there were 21 beds in total. Other resources were a bathroom with one large bath and one sit-up bath, and a sluice area with bedpan washer, cubicle shower and waste disposal area. Staff had access to a separate locked toilet on the main hospital corridor a few feet away from the ward.

The staff

The staff, whom I refer to throughout by pseudonyms, were led by a ward sister I shall call Caroline. There were seven staff nurses, one of which was permanently on night duty. Other staff nurses rotated to night duty approximately every three months. The nursing staff were perhaps slightly unusual in one respect at least, as they were generally quite highly qualified academically. Two of the staff nurses possessed degrees and two more were pursuing degree-level work. Of eight students who were on or came to the ward during my fieldwork, two had degrees and one was a qualified teacher. Of those with degrees, none were in nursing. The two part time students were studying nursing subjects, however. During my fieldwork period three of the total of sixteen nursing staff with whom I had substantial contact were male. I give brief details of the role and position of respondents in the text where it is of relevance. I have, however, kept biographical pictures to a minimum as an aid to anonymity. I had relatively little contact with medical staff during my fieldwork. I introduced myself to doctors as occasion demanded, and do not feel that I arose undue feelings of suspicion. They generally seemed comfortable with the notion of nurse researchers. I sometimes attended ward rounds where nursing staff would normally have done so, but did not take up the offer when occasionally people assumed that as a researcher this would be where my interests lay. As a matter of information however, five consultants routinely attended the ward and others would attend emergency admissions who were lodgers. Domestic staff were employed by an outside contractor and seemed to play little part in ward activity except in terms of their tight remit to clean and tidy the ward. Consequently my interactions with them were brief and of an instrumental type.

Ward organisation

The ward work was explicitly organised on an team nursing basis. That is to say, that staff nurses and students were allocated every two weeks to one of two teams, A or B. In most cases and especially until the evening, nurses worked primarily with the patients on their side (or team) of the ward. The allocation was changed every two weeks because staff had found that one side always seemed to be harder than the other. This manoeuvre also varied experience for students whilst allowing them a good spell to get to know many of their patients.

Care planning

The night staff would routinely hand over to almost all the day staff in a short report. Later after breakfasts were given to those patients who seemed ready and willing, a more detailed report was given by the team leader to their own team. Whilst the team leader was often a staff nurse, sometimes new students were given experience in running through the nursing process Kardex, with supplementary information being offered by the more experienced staff. First year students at first felt very worried by this, but soon seemed to gain in confidence, and it was an aspect of their development of which they were happy to boast at coffee time to their colleagues on other wards. As the day went by staff would help on the other side if a team was clearly struggling, or if help was required with a very heavy patient.

Overall atmosphere

According to the handout designed for student nurses and provided to me by the sister when I arrived, the ward staff aimed to provide 'a friendly, relaxed environment which facilitates learning and the production of high standards of care.' It was no part of my remit to attempt to evaluate this learning climate as others have done (Orton, 1981: Smith, 1992). I merely offer an opinion, that despite the persistence of some clear status boundaries, the ward had, in comparison to many, a relaxed atmosphere in which most senior staff were seen as fairly approachable by students. Students themselves made this very clear to me. I will now examine in more detail some of the key moral questions that I believe I faced in conducting the study in this setting.

Ethical issues

Ethical issues have been insufficiently addressed in both the teaching and practice of research. In research reports there is of course a balance to be struck. As Dingwall (1980) argues, there are limitations to conventional professional self-regulation whereby it has to some extent been assumed that ethnographers are by definition 'good people'. Such an approach has led in some cases to dubious moral conduct with little or no articulated moral justification. I argue that some rationale should be offered by researchers of their approach, especially where that approach might reasonably provoke controversy.

In *A Silent Conspiracy?: Some Ethical Issues in Participant Observation in Nursing Research* (Johnson, 1992) I discuss a number of key issues which ought to be considered by investigators in observer roles in clinical areas. In particular I discuss motives for research activity, the notion of privacy of informants, and the question of informed consent. I also discuss the question of deception in covert research activity as exemplified in a study by Mary Knight and David Field (Field, 1989). I conclude by arguing that covert research activity in a ward and specifically studying the dying and the people who care for them would normally require great justification, and certainly more than Dr. Field provides in his popular book. Indeed, I argue that all covert research activity would need more than the merely technical justifications such as "..communication and general behaviour were natural and normal" (Field, 1989:35).

In the paper I address perspectives such as *utilitarianism* and the *human rights* which may be utilised in evaluating the moral conduct (or intended conduct) of researchers. It is not my intention here to repeat the arguments rehearsed in that paper, but to address the key issues as they affected my own study and to present a justification of my own position.

Motive

As I explain in the introduction my wish to undertake clinical research fits well with my role as an academic in a university. Clinical contact helps me to maintain a degree of credibility if not expertise in clinical matters. The pursuit of academic qualifications or research publications can imply using respondents as means to an end rather than as an end in themselves. I suggest, however, that methods such as overt participant observation go some way to redressing the balance. True participants have an opportunity to bargain for data, that is, they have something to offer respondents which is worth having. I undertook a good deal of physical and emotional labour during my time in the clinical area as may be evident from my later discussions of the data I obtained. I was also able to act to some extent as a resource to staff who wanted to discuss career development and sometimes other issues. I asked most of my respondents what it was like having me 'on their backs', so to speak. Invariably they suggested that they soon got used to me and saw me as a greater help than a hindrance. Of course, whilst they might be expected to say this to me, many were fairly experienced and assertive, and some of these interviews were done after I had finished working in the setting and so it seems fair to assume that they were speaking honestly.

I am still left with a feeling that, despite the help I may have been able to offer, a better approach might have been to do the study from a more clearly action research perspective. Greenwood (1984) and Webb (1989) have put forward vigorous cases for action research as a solution to this and other problems of research justification, and I would certainly seriously consider this kind of approach in the future. More recently I have myself argued that action research from a humanistic perspective renders motive explicit to participants in the research and moves research activity very fruitfully in a mutually beneficial direction (Johnson, 1997).

Informed consent

David Field (1989) has, such as it is, the protection of a long tradition of covert research in sociology to justify his deception of the dying, their relatives, their nurses and others in the collection of his data. Even more, his study has dated by some 15 years now since its data was collected. Whilst I might hope that either covert research would decrease or its justification improve, I find this sadly is not always the case. A study by a nurse as recently published as December 1996 (Clark, 1996a, 1996b) seems to me to take an approach beyond understanding.

Clark clearly set out to collect data which would contradict claims made by a secure mental health unit about the style of care provided. In this, Clark admits that he had hypotheses which pre-existed the data collection. He argues that the unit 'publicly declared itself a therapeutic community' a claim which Clark argues 'seemed unlikely given that the unit consisted of a locked ward populated by residents who were offenders' (1996a: 37). In order to refute their claims, Clark (who seems otherwise to be a lecturer) gained a position as a paid nursing auxiliary for a six week period and collected data by chatting to colleagues and 'eavesdropping'. In one of the two publications relating to this work, Clark suggests that:

...subjects were aware that observations were being carried out even if they were not always aware that they were being observed. Such

43

eavesdropping was always within sight of relevant subjects and only clandestine in as much as they might have though I was really reading a newspaper when I was actually just pretending (1996a: p38).

Whilst it may be that in some cases covert observation is justifiable, I suggest that Clark fails to meet any such position. First, being covert was probably unnecessary to analyse the ward organisation style. It is highly unlikely that the people on the unit could or would have re-oriented their whole system of care just because they had an ethnographer, however openly, in their midst. Second, however much he may feel to the contrary, he has inevitably collected data from, and therefore deceived, not only his colleagues but also the clients in the unit. Clark chooses to distinguish his work as an ethnography, but fails totally to recognise the point that thereby it should be an analysis of the whole culture of the setting which, inevitably, includes clients. Third, Clark has confused the theoretical implausibility of gaining total and *completely* informed consent with the practical convenience to himself of gaining none at all. Not only has Clark deceived his clients and nursing colleagues on the unit he studied (and with what real gain?) it seems to me that he has deceived himself about the natures of ethnography and informed consent into the bargain.

I repeat that covert research ought not to be excluded absolutely from consideration, but that its nature, purpose and justification should be rather more coherent than I find with either Field (1989) or most recently Clark (1996 a and b). As for my own study reported here, I gained permission to approach the staff on Howarth ward through the Health Authority Ethics Committee, the Director of Nursing of the Unit and written authority to practise from the Chief Nurse. I then approached the ward sister, who knew that I had the authorisation of these persons in authority. It is difficult to judge whether, having gained permission to proceed from these senior agencies, the ward staff would then feel intimidated to comply. I did however insist on speaking to the staff each day when I arrived until the majority of them knew who I was and why I was there. I explained that I am a nurse and also now a teacher of nurse teachers in higher education. I said that my aim was to examine how nurses and others deal with 'moral decisions', which was as much as I myself knew. I stressed that they could ask me any questions and that I would answer them fully, and that I would terminate the study if they felt uncomfortable with my presence.

As new nurses arrived I would brief them, but commonly their colleagues had put them in the picture beforehand. Roth (1962) suggests that in settings like hospitals it is never possible to get informed consent from all from whom data might be collected (Clark's argument for *ignoring* informed consent!). Many people visit the area and it is not practical to

44

give everybody the briefing and get their permission to quote the comment they made when they came into the ward office. This is especially true of patients, some of whom are too ill to have the whole idea explained. Any comfort which can be obtained in the notion that patients who come to a teaching hospital can expect to be the subject of teaching and research is slight indeed.

Rather, what Williams (1989) describes as 'practical ethics' have to come into play. Decisions are made about what to tell people in the light of their incapacity and the practicality of doing so. Rules and codes are relatively unhelpful. I wore a badge which said *nurse researcher* but in many cases I was perceived as an ordinary member of staff and so most of my patient informants did not give explicit permission to me to utilise data. Seen from a consequentialist position, the outcome of my approach was no different from that of Field (1989), whose reliance on data covertly obtained I criticise (Johnson, 1992). We have both collected and reported data from people who, for whatever different reasons, have not given informed consent.

To return to pragmatism, if not utilitarianism, for some justification, I suggest the following. To attempt reasonably to give information about the research to all those for whom this is possible reduces the number of those to whom, for good reasons, it is not practical to do so. Deliberately to deceive even those who might have been able to benefit from the knowledge that research is being done must be worse. Williams' (1989) point about practical ethics, that rules and codes are useless when confronted with live dilemmas in the social setting is very valid, especially within a reflexive framework in which researchers disclose those areas where they feel troubled by the moral status of their conduct. Dingwall, (1977), Williams, (1989), James (1986) and Webb (1989) have begun to set new standards of reflexive writing in the matter of practical research ethics which are helpful in a way in which formalised codes of conduct, for example that of the Royal College of Nursing (1977) are not.

Intervention

Participant observation in the role of a qualified nurse implies that intervention is the norm, that is to say that as a nurse I undertook those activities which seemed professionally sensible at the time. By intervention here however, I mean to discuss those deliberate actions which go beyond or even contravene the norms of ward behaviour in order to protect the perceived interests of one or more persons (usually patients).

Deciding when and how to intervene to improve the lives of respondents, especially clients, has long troubled researchers in health settings, but it has been little discussed. In *Observations on the neglected concept of intervention in nursing research* (Johnson, 1997) I develop more fully some of the points I touch upon here, analysing the issues as they confront both positivistic and naturalistic researchers. Here, however I will focus briefly on issues in this study.

This too is a case of practical ethics since, as Dingwall (1980) suggests, there is the risk of witnessing poor practice and thus allowing informants to believe that the researcher shares acceptance of this behaviour. He argues that, particularly where the researcher holds a professional qualification for the field under study (such as nursing), failure to intervene could be personally compromising.

On the other hand, as I have found as a teacher in clinical areas, excessively 'correct' behaviour is not seen to be credible or maintainable over long periods and can break down trust painstakingly obtained. For example there is a professional norm that soiled tissues, clothes and sheets are not put on the floor but directly into a special bag. The principles of hygiene which this upholds are self-evident even if actual deleterious consequences to clients through some supposed route of cross infection are remote. Under difficult conditions of cleaning leakage of faecal material from a patient who had just come out of the bath in a lifting device, one of my student nurse co-participants put the tissues on the floor. In a perfect world she would have had a soiled dressings bag ready. She did not have gloves on either, which both for aesthetic and hygienic reasons is also the norm. Intervention here, by me as a qualified nurse, would have meant preventing or stopping the inappropriate activity, and discussing the 'right way'. Unfortunately it is not that easy. The transgression seemed to me to be fairly minor: floors can be cleaned. If anything, what she did protected the client's dignity a little by not making a fuss of the leak rather than rushing for gloves and bags. I felt that she knew the 'rules'. She had elected to break them in those particular circumstances, and the behaviour was not in my view 'dangerous'. The look we gave each other communicated all these things, and the sense that she did not need to be told that being better prepared next time would help.

This is an example of a small as opposed to a big dilemma where intervention (or non-intervention) would be much harder to decide upon. I had a general policy that if I witnessed anything resembling negligent or unsafe conduct then I would compromise my position as a researcher and take the necessary action in patients' interests. This of course is at the other extreme, but a good deal of what the ethnographer sees is conduct which is not bad but which could possibly be better.

In one circumstance I was uncomfortable because an elderly and very debilitated patient seemed to be having uncomfortable investigations which, if his own clear wishes had been noted, he would not have had.

Intervention here would have meant assuming a direct patient advocate role in opposition to both medical staff and relatives. (I discuss the situation at greater length later). I can try to justify to myself that not being on the staff meant I was not responsible. Harris (1985) argues persuasively, however, that on such questions, status or professional role have no legitimate bearing. People have the same responsibility to right wrongs whatever their contractual position. I have no defence against this morally persuasive consequentialist position except to plead the weakness derived from my own personal and professional socialisation.

Dingwall (1980) in his discussion of the *prevailing motive of ethnography* also supports my position, though I am far from happy with this as a rationale:

> In theory, the researcher is neither a journalist nor a crusader with a mandate to titillate or moralise. (His) main thrust is to report the 'good reasons' which subjects adduce to account for their actions and, thereby, to furnish the context within which their conduct, however objectionable, becomes rational. (Dingwall, 1980:881)

With this we return to some form of contextual ethical decision model on whether to intervene. What is important is that such problems are openly discussed so that research supervisors and colleagues both in the setting and subsequently can offer some kind of reasoned opinion upon researcher conduct.

Summary

In this section I have outlined my negotiation of access to the setting I call Howarth Ward and discussed some of the concerns I had in relation to the moral questions I faced and the positions I had in mind as justification. Issues of greatest concern to me were informed consent and the practical impossibility of obtaining it from everyone, and researcher intervention both in serious and in much less serious matters. I am mindful of the contextual nature of much decision-making on moral questions, to which Williams (1989) draws special attention as a nurse and ethnographer.

5 Good and bad patients: a review in depth

As was planning to use grounded theory, I avoided too substantial an immersion in the literature until after the main fieldwork. However, a considerable literature does exist and I had some knowledge of key papers such as that by Kelly and May (1982). As the initial analysis of data clearly showed that the phenomenon of social judgement of persons was of major interest, I have attempted to introduce the topic by critically reviewing a small selection of the more influential papers in the area.

'Good and bad' patients literature

This review is organised in broadly chronological order since part of my intention is to show how researchers in this area have varied in their grasp of the underlying perspectives of the research approaches they use. My particular focus has been to examine the developing methods and research perspectives of previous work, and I will place less emphasis upon 'findings' at this point. Where such findings are important to compare or contrast with my own they are incorporated into the relevant sections of this text. Also I am writing explicitly from an interactionist perspective, and this will flavour my comments about previous work.

Michael Kelly and David May wrote a very comprehensive review of the 'good and bad patients' literature in 1982. They list virtually all work which had been done until that date, and classify it generally into themes. They then deliver a strong attack on much of the work but do so having considered most papers together so that the consideration of individual articles is minimal. Indeed whilst their model of the literature review has much to commend it, I would argue that sometimes it is better to examine less work in greater detail than they found possible in their article. Rather than repeat their work here I intend to select individual papers and illustrate their importance in the wider scheme of things. I have included work from Britain and some from both the USA and Australia.

The perception that some patients are seen by staff as good and some bad is far from new. In a study of cultural components in response to pain in American citizens, Zborowski (1952) had noted the fact that some patients desired to seek the approval of staff, and particularly that they did not want to be 'nuisances'.

As an in-service training director for nursing staff, Miriam Ritvo (1963) seems to have 'interviewed' more than 1000 nursing personnel, and obtained written responses from 500 more. Her open question 'What is a good patient?' elicited a range of behaviours or qualities of which co-operative, appreciative, accepting own illness and accepting prescribed treatment were the most popular of a wide range of responses. 'Bad' patients were those who, among other traits, were demanding and unreasonable.

It seems that Ritvo used notes from her general discussions with staff on training sessions, often in groups, as the interview data. It is not clear whether respondents knew they were participants in research activity, but the determination to include such large numbers of respondents does at least ensure anonymity for individuals if not the institutions, which are more easily identified. Written in a journal not explicitly designed for research publications, and with only the one reference, to Zborowski, this is nevertheless an interesting early attempt to undertake an analysis. Once analysed for traits, these were counted and presented as percentages. Ritvo offers some tentative explanations of her data. In those cases of nurses who denied that they ever label a patient (18%), she asks whether these nurses might be more *intuitive* or better *trained in human relations skills* than other nurses covered by the survey. As might be expected from a training associate at Boston University Human Relations Center, Mrs. Ritvo concludes her study by making a case for greater emphasis on this type of training in basic and in-service programmes. This, she argues, might be:

> ...to eliminate the necessity for a patient to become "good" or "bad" and to remove the burden from the ill person of the need to be popular at a time when (he) may feel (himself) 'least likely to succeed' (p81)

Given that this study predates the major Royal College of Nursing (UK) research programme which commenced in 1969 and which included the influential *The unpopular patient* by Felicity Stockwell (1972), Ritvo's (1963) paper deserves some attention.

A trait theory?

A good example of a largely prescriptive paper, but which summarises some key elements of the *traits theory* of goodness and badness is the work of Papper (1970). An editorial in the *Journal of Chronic Diseases* (and having been presented previously at a medical intern's banquet!), the paper attempts to remind physicians that despite the Hippocratic Oath they may regard some patients as undesirable. Papper suggests, based I assume upon his clinical experience since he offers no data, that there are five categories of undesirable patient. Social undesirability he takes to be being alcoholic, aged, dirty, uneducated or very poor. His second category, attitudinal undesirability, includes being ungrateful, wanting to know too much, and 'thinking he knows so much'. Papper suggests that these latter traits imply something less than total faith in the physician, and goes on to point out that those patients who really do know too much (such as physicians as patients) also constitute difficulty for the physician. Papper locates the reason for undesirability here in patients' failure to meet physicians' expectations and needs. He does not elaborate about these needs, but I assume it is the physician's need not to be questioned and not to be contradicted.

Papper argues that patients may be undesirable on physical grounds such as the absence of physical illness, or the presence of illness which shows the physician's initial diagnosis to be in error. Included in this third category of undesirability are 'lack of response to good treatment', chronic illness, malignant illness and 'ordinary illness' such as stroke.

These sorts of categories appear frequently in subsequent literature and are clearly located in permanent or semi permanent features or traits of patients. Papper's last two categories briefly acknowledge factors external to the patient. These he calls 'circumstantial undesirability' and 'distraction undesirability'. The former is that in which the physician forms a bad impression because, for example, the consultation took place in a busy and overcrowded clinic. The latter, the fifth and final category, is one in which the doctor sees the patient as undesirable because 'he' does not fit with the interests and orientation of the times. Here Papper principally draws attention to the physician's research priorities in which patients seem uninteresting if they are not valuable as research subjects. In his conclusion Papper argues that self-discipline might help to prevent undesirable labels being attached to patients, and stresses the point that in relation to research activity the physician's first duty is to the individual patient, who must have a higher priority than any other consideration.

Papper's views are consistent with the predominantly *patient traits* explanations which have been and still are popular and to which he arguably makes a limited contribution. His paper, written by an experienced and senior physician, must be classified as prescriptive.

Social processes?

In 1972 the influential sociologist Julius Roth published a paper on the 'moral evaluation' and control of the clientele of a hospital emergency service. (Note: Roth's term moral evaluation may be taken to mean what I now term social judgement for reasons I explain in detail later. Broadly speaking a member of the Chicago School of sociology and allied to an interpretive approach, Roth and his colleagues naturally used participant observation and informal interviews to collect data in six accident and emergency departments. He suggests that work on the *moral evaluation* of clients had previously concentrated upon the mentally ill, such as that by Goffman (1968), and others.

This was, he argues, because the treatment and diagnosis of mental illness was seen to be technologically deficient, or more open to alternative explanation, than medical illness. The label *mentally ill* is more easily seen as a social construction, defined in relation to a culture and a time, than medical illness which is arguably more 'scientific' and thus more reliably identified. However, Roth complains that this focus upon the mentally ill as those most likely to have their behaviour categorised as morally reprehensible or deviant, has ignored the obvious fact that persons with straightforward medical diseases are also capable of being morally evaluated (or socially judged), that is seen as good or bad. As Roth notes:

> ...the diagnosis and treatment of mental illness and the 'care' of mental patients are not unique in incorporating moral judgements of the clientele, but are obvious examples of a more general phenomenon which exists no matter what the historical development or the present state of the technology. (p839)

He goes on to remind us that Glaser and Strauss (1964) had drawn attention to the phenomenon indirectly with their paper on the *social loss* or social worth of dying patients. As with Glaser and Strauss, Roth attempts to examine the phenomenon of labelling and moral evaluation in terms of social processes rather than in terms of traits which patients or their carers possess. Roth points out that the first person dealing with a new client, such as the admitting nurse or clerk, can have a good deal of influence in applying judgmental label which then can govern future care. Making his case in some detail, he argues that there are broadly two types of evaluations that are carried out. The first is the application of wider societal conceptions of moral worth, for example that 'drunks' and women with a presumed promiscuous sexual history are less deserving of treatment. The second relates to the staff's conceptions of their work roles:

> Every worker has a notion of what demands are appropriate to (the) position. When demands fall outside that boundary (the worker) feels that the claim is illegitimate. (Roth, 1972:845)

Roth gives examples which show that what the worker does about this depends upon power to control the behaviour of others and the power to select clientele. On this latter point Roth suggests that if selection is impossible, then the tactic of avoidance becomes the norm. He suggests that there are sanctions which staff apply to 'bad' patients, but that these amount more to 'training' the clients to be 'good' than punishments. By good he means clients who fit the criteria for legitimate demands for services, and Roth gives examples of how patients are kept waiting, a strategy which it is difficult for clients to challenge because of the complexity and busyness of hospitals.

Roth acknowledges some of the limitations of his formulations and urges that more research of this nature be undertaken in a variety of settings. As it happens he seems to have provoked quite an outcrop of studies of emergency (casualty) departments as will become clear. Where his paper seems to be weakest is in the assumption that because he and his colleagues 'were there', his observations and conclusions are to be taken on trust. He uses data only sparingly in the nature of examples, and so it is difficult to evaluate the rigour of his analysis. This is true of much research in this tradition and applies equally to later papers by sociologists and may be substantially to do with the need for economies of space in journals. Roth fails to escape completely from the notion that traits are primarily the origin of social judgement, focusing as he does upon 'drunks' and 'pelvic inflammatory disease' as sources of negative evaluation. However he certainly re-orientates theoretical notions of unpopularity toward a dynamic and complex social process involving concepts like power.

Stockwell's approach

There is a very much quoted British study by Felicity Stockwell published in 1972 and which was undertaken as part of the wider *Study of Nursing Care* series. This series of twelve studies was funded by the Department of Health and Social Security and administered by the Royal College of Nursing. The overall aim of the project was to develop criteria of quality of care. It is probably fair to say that all the studies were located within a broadly positivist perspective. That is to say they generally attempted to quantify variables and the relationships between them. Studies investigating psychological phenomena such as student nurses' anxiety (Birch 1975) would use questionnaires to relate biographical and psychological variables and to attempt to draw conclusions. Where observation of the social world did occur this generally used a predetermined checklist or structured observation sheet (e.g. Cormack, 1976). Where qualitative data became available this was generally seen as second order data, only of value in support of other quantified aspects (see for example Lelean, 1973).

It is impossible to dispute the value of these early British attempts to collect systematic information about nursing. The studies have become widely available and been a part of the slow but sure development of interest in a research base upon which to base nursing actions. However, in retrospect it is possible to speculate upon the influence these studies have had in the promulgation of a quantification emphasis in nursing research. The Government funding which supported the studies was a pull in a policy-oriented and quantitative direction, since it is assumed that policy is more easily justified by evidence in figures. Another influence, apart from the wider attempt to mimic the more established social and behavioural and medical sciences, may have been the academic direction of the early project directors, notably Jean McFarlane, whose own Masters' thesis was published in part as *The Proper Study of the Nurse* (1971) and was written from a management perspective. Later, from her key position in the nursing establishment Jean, later Professor the Baroness McFarlane of Llandaff was increasingly to endorse ethnographic approaches such as that by Sylvia Kappeli (1984) whom she supervised.

McFarlane, as she points out in the preface to a 1984 reprinted edition of Felicity Stockwell's well-known *The unpopular patient*, supervised this work too. The study begins with an attempt to test (in particular) the hypothesis that there are observable and measurable differences in the nursing care given to popular and unpopular patients. It then ends with an attempt to 'generate theory'. Stockwell clearly began by attempting to produce and use an instrument which would identify and measure 'patient unpopularity'.

Whilst she felt that she had some success in producing an instrument which would discriminate in ranking terms, eventually the quantitative aspect of the study founders. Page 25 makes clear in a summary the inadequacy of the quantitative part of the study:

...there was evidence to suggest that foreign patients, those in hospital for more than three months and those with more than three months' previous experience of hospital, and those with some kind of defect, figured significantly in the unpopular group. It also appeared that patients with a psychiatric diagnosis (including..suicide attempt) were more likely to be found unpopular than popular, although it was not possible to submit this particular factor to significance tests, as questions on it had not been included in the particulars collected about the patients. (Stockwell, 1972, reprint 1984:25)

This gives a flavour of the failure of the attempt to give percentage scores to patients' popularity in order realistically to determine what were and were not the 'causal variables'. The causal variables were from the beginning assumed to be wholly patient related. Using the hindsight possible in a reprinted edition, both Stockwell and McFarlane acknowledge some likely weaknesses of the study in a general way, but they point out that not only did the study draw 'dramatic attention to the inadequacies of nurse-patient interaction' (p3) but it 'pioneered new ground in research design and method' (also p3). This it certainly did, if not in elegance, then as an example of retrieval of a worthwhile project by shifting perspective: in this case from quantitative to qualitative. The second half of the work is devoted to a quasi-ethnographic description of 'life in four wards' as it affected the popular and the unpopular. Although the aim was to use the constant comparative analytic method of Glaser and Strauss (1967), judged against more recent and perhaps more rigorous theory-generating studies the account is descriptive rather than explanatory. Nevertheless there is much rich 'naturalistic' data and the conclusion that Stockwell and possibly McFarlane were at their most comfortable using this approach is inescapable.

Throughout the study, both in the quantified elements and in the observation study Stockwell (being a nurse) evidently chose to be non-participant, even to the extent of trying to find a nurse for a patient who needed one. The study is written, as are many even today, as if it were done by someone else, the researcher. This part of the account addresses issues such as the sanctions that she perceived nurses to use in the control of unacceptable behaviour, such as ignoring the patient, forgetting patients' requests, enforcing rules and using sarcasm. I am bound now to wonder whether Stockwell was comfortable with this objective approach.

Lorber's survey

Judith Lorber (1975) undertook a small but widely quoted study in a New York 'bedroom borough'. She asked 103 routine surgical patients to respond, on a Likert type scale of agreement and disagreement, to six statements. (Examples of which are 'the sicker a patient is the more

54

attention he or she can expect from the doctors and the nurses, and the best thing to do in hospital is to keep quiet and do what you're told.) (p.216)

From the responses, Lorber categorised patients on a continuum from conformity to deviance. Other data were collected by interviews which took place just before discharge and patients were asked whether they had "refused to follow a doctor's or a nurse's order or complained about one". (It is not clear whether this would be a complaint about the nurse or doctor or about their order). Lorber also collected data from staff by self-administered questionnaire.

She draws a number of conclusions from her data, which generally reflect the notion that patients who were no trouble to the staff were good patients and those who were troublesome were likely to be bad. She argues that 'the best predictors' of conforming and deviant attitudes toward the hospital patient role were age and education. That is, the younger and/or the better educated patients were more likely to be non-compliant, and as a consequence labelled as bad. She further argues that from the doctors' and nurses' points of view, ease of management was "the basic criterion for a label of a good patient" (p220).

Lorber had previously been a colleague of the eminent Eliot Freidson whose theoretical perspective in all his main work is interpretive sociology (see Freidson, 1970). Lorber herself in this paper seems to refer most to workers in this tradition (including Freidson's book), but it is clear that in this paper at least she is prepared to collect her data and offer explanations in primarily quantitative and Functionalist terms. Her highly structured questionnaire/interview clearly presupposes a definitive theory of conformity in surgical patients and its associated causal variables, e.g. age and education. She makes little attempt to gain access to the patients' experience of the situation or to imagine any factors other than patient behaviour and patients' attitudes which might influence the social definition of the good or problem patient.

Lorber offers an account of consequences which may befall patients labelled as troublesome. Some patients were given tranquillisers, and others who do not respond to this were referred to a psychiatrist which, she argues, has 'the most potentially momentous consequences' (p223). For various reasons, such as the fall into disfavour of many sedatives (e.g. Diazepam) and the expense and low availability of psychiatric referrals in the UK. these strategies seem particularly mismatched with the current British context. From my point of view, Lorber's paper contains its most useful discussion in its examination of the findings and insights offered by other papers notably, as I have mentioned, by qualitative sociologists like Roth and Glaser and Strauss. Even seen strictly in terms of an exploratory social survey accepting and using the methods of such survey work (e.g.

Moser and Kalton, 1971) the paper has elemental flaws and draws conclusions beyond the data such as in her penultimate paragraph:

> Such problem patients, in this study, were tranquillised, sometimes discharged early, and, in one case, referred to a psychiatrist... (p224)

and her final remarks:

> Thus, the consequences of deliberate deviance in the general hospital can be medical neglect or a stigmatizing label, while conformity to good-patient norms is usually a return home with only a surgical scar. (p224)

These are powerful conclusions to be drawn from asking patients (who are still in hospital) six Likert scale questions. She provides, so far as I can see, no evidence for 'medical neglect' in her account of her study. Despite the assertion of Kelly and May (1982) that Lorber's paper is one of only a few they find not guilty of 'analytic individualism', I am less convinced. I find that whilst broadly sympathetic to the interpretive perspective, Lorber's assumptions about individual behaviour, attitudes and other variables like age and education are indeed located in a patients' traits explanation of unpopularity. She does acknowledge to a greater degree than other, even much later work, that power is a key concept in such explanations. However her design, execution and the report of the study lend little weight to her theoretical suggestions.

'Rubbish' in casualty?

Roth's naturalistic lead and clearly interpretive approach was developed in the United Kingdom by an influential paper by Jeffery (1979). He used several months' participant observation in the increasingly popular research area of casualty departments as his data-base. Here, Jeffery identified two broad categories into which medical staff placed their clients. These were 'good or interesting', which name already implies the reason they are seen to be 'good', and 'bad or rubbish'. Jeffery argues that some patients become defined as good because they allow medical staff to practise skills necessary for passing their examinations, they allow staff to practise their chosen speciality, and they test the skills and maturity of the staff. Thus such patients, in the casualty setting at least, were those who were not routine and who were of interest from a medical point of view.

'Rubbish' was defined as those patients who in some way broke one or more of the following neo Parsonian obligations or rules:

1. They must not be responsible for their illness or for getting better.
2. Patients should be rendered unable to carry out their normal activities by the complaint with which they report to casualty.
3. They should see the illness as undesirable.
4. Patients should co-operate with medical staff in wanting to get well.

Reed and Bond (1986), Dingwall and Murray (1983) and Jeffery himself all drew attention to the roots of this explanation in the Parsonian (1951) concept of the *sick role* in which the above four rules are approximately those which a person normally adheres to in order to sustain the functional therapeutic relationship with the doctor. According to Dingwall and Murray (1983), Jeffrey's analysis fails to account for a large category of patients which they found to be anonymous or 'ordinary', that is neither good nor bad. The paper does however represent an early important British study of the notion of social judgement of clients and later papers have built on his ideas, as I shall show.

Analysing stereotypes

A study by Worsley (1980) about whom we know only that he or she works in the *Division of Human Nutrition, C.S.I.R.O.* in Adelaide Australia, analysed 79 (all female) student nurses' stereotypes of 'liked' and 'disliked' patients at a Melbourne general hospital. Worsley obtained qualitative data in written form in response to a request to the students to describe the patients they both liked and disliked most in their recent ward experience. The data were then analysed for factors both intuitively and quantitatively by computer. Factors relating positively or negatively to 'the favourite patient' for example were named and interpreted mostly as follows:

- Friendliness-co-operation
- Anxiety-depression
- Aggression-noncooperation
- Annoyingness-dirtiness
- Apparent age
- Helplessness
- Demandingness

The computerised statistical analysis is complex. However, Worsley explains its relevance to the interpretation of findings and the study is a good example of the perceived need to quantify and to apply inferential statistical methods to possibly rich qualitative data. Given the relative potency of traits or individualised explanations of good and bad patients which continues yet, the study aims to ascribe degrees of importance and weight to the factors or variables within the traits theory which supposedly predict unpopularity. I risk oversimplification here but in principle the results indicate that a theory of popularity/unpopularity should be as follows:

For the favourite patient, 'friendly co-operation' dominated the factor structure, whilst 'emotional distress' played a similar role in the disliked patient analysis. Worsley accepts some limitations of the work which are also taken to be recommendations for further study. The concept of 'self-fulfilling prophecy' is mentioned, which has been seen as a feature of the more 'interpretive' labelling theory and suggests that the relationship of nurses' stereotypes to overt behaviour would be worthy of examination. Worsley suggests that aggregating nurses' views and stereotypes as a mean score (as was done) may have problems in that individual nurses may have differing views.

Overall, and with her psychometric testing perspective firmly in mind, Worsley's study is a further contribution to what I term the trait theory of social judgement of patients by staff. Whilst she uncritically quotes Goffman's (1959) *Presentation of Self in Everyday Life* in the first sentence of the paper it is difficult to see in what way, other than brief mention of self-fulfilling prophecies, the study is influenced by his theoretical orientation.

I have argued that Roth's (1972) work in the USA. made some progress in refocusing the discussion of good and bad patients upon the staff involved in the labelling and upon social processes rather than 'patients' attributes'. With only a few notable exceptions it was to continue to be professional sociologists rather than nurses who would recognise the importance of a process perspective in understanding social phenomena in health care delivery and social judgement of clients in particular.

'Dirty work'

The British sociologist Phil Strong (1980) drew upon Everett Hughes' sociology of work to identify and extend the analysis of 'dirty work'. Strong conducted informal interviews with a group of Scottish General Practitioners. Discussing the case of alcoholics, Strong immediately draws attention to the differing explanations which have been offered for this group of patients being seen as 'dirty work'. Quoting from Hughes' original contribution Strong defines dirty work as:

> ...tasks ...considered nuisances and impositions or even dirty work - physically, socially or morally beneath the dignity of the profession. (Strong, 1980:24)

Although by concentrating upon *alcoholics* as a group Strong necessarily assumes that this trait is important as a determinant of professionals' reactions, he goes well beyond naive suggestions that alcoholics, as a group, constitute a single category. He first of all explores competing explanations of generalised medical distaste for alcoholics all of which refocus interest in the doctor rather than assuming it is patient traits which best explain the phenomenon. Among these he lists ignorance of the medical possibilities for treatment and the idea that authoritarian doctors will dislike alcoholics more. Other previous explanations he includes are the placing of blame upon the patient to cover up the doctor's lack of motivation and expertise in such cases, and the idea that greater social distance between client and professional means greater unpopularity. Finally he alludes to a theory that general social attitudes are moving from a 'moral theory of alcoholic behaviour' to a medical explanation and that once versed in the new approach doctors will not see treating the disorder as dirty work.

Strong tentatively rejects these ideas, arguing that the preceding explanations can be summarised as ignorance and prejudice on the part of the doctor and do not account for other and quite rational grounds for the medical profession's avoidance of alcoholics. In some detail, and with examples from his acknowledged limited data, Strong sets forth a counter-explanation of medical avoidance. In summary he argues that the dislike felt by general practitioners for handling alcoholics was based, at least in part, on highly rational grounds. Alcoholics did not satisfy any of the ordinary assumptions upon which the therapeutic relationship was usually based. The doctors had neither cures nor special knowledge of the problem, and many alcoholics would not define their drinking as problematic. In Strong's own words:

> Thus, alcoholism was a messy business in which there was often little to be gained by any active medical intervention. This fundamental dysjunction with the standard role-relationship seems a more plausible account of why alcoholics should be dirty work than that of traditional morality or faulty education. (p 42-43)

In his account Strong is very aware of the limitations of his data but offers general hypotheses for consideration which modify existing notions of doctors' perceptions of alcoholics. Strong's (1980) work also illustrates a point about the intellectual and professional maturity of the work of British interpretive sociologists above that of work published by nurses. There is full acknowledgement of potential criticisms, there is a good attempt to avoid purely reductive or individualised explanations of social phenomena, and the work is written in the perfectly natural first person singular so that the opinions and responsibility for them are not disguised as those of some other totally dispassionate scientist. This latter point is elaborated by Webb (1992) and by Porter (1993) in their separate critiques of the stylistic limitations of some of the main nursing journals and their editorial advisors.

Kelly and May's interactionist critique

I have briefly acknowledged the influential paper by Michael Kelly and David May (1982) in which they list all the main publications on 'good and bad patients' to that date. They offer a strong criticism of most of the work suggesting, from their interactionist perspective, that most of the studies are:

> ...deficient from an empirical, a methodological, an epistemological and a theoretical point of view. (p147)

Generally their thesis, the main thrust of which I will show that I accept, is that most of the studies locate discussion of and research into good and bad patients in the assumption that it is necessarily patient characteristics that are the chief determinant of the reception of such labels and their consequences. Kelly and May note that the themes which have emerged in the literature are first of all the disease or illness the patient suffered. Predictors of unpopularity are exemplified by being confused, having a terminal illness, and being incontinent. Illnesses associated with popularity were said to be those in which dramatic recoveries are made or those which test particular clinical skills. Kelly and May discuss the rather less consistent views about patient behaviour and popularity, in which the common determinant of a bad label is deviant or rule-breaking behaviour, such as non-conformity to medical regime. Some traits are said to have both good and bad effects, such as the degree of patient dependency upon staff. Patients can be too dependent or not dependent enough (too independent), and it is to examine this sort of ambiguity that Kelly and May argue for a change of focus in 'good and bad' patient research. Work on the attitudes of patients, their perceived intelligence, other biographical and social variables such as social class and education is also reviewed and the same broad conclusions drawn.

Almost all previous work in the area is heavily criticised by Kelly and May on three main counts. First, that on empirical grounds many studies are 'contradictory and inconsistent', that is, they report opposite or differing findings in examination of the same variables. Whilst interpretive researchers (such as ethnographers) make little claim to generalisability of findings, most of the work that Kelly and May review is quantitative and therefore uses inferential statistics in support of its conclusions. It is thus quite reasonable, they argue, to judge this work by the canons of scientific research, such as repeatability in differing settings. By these standards the findings are often equivocal.

They then attack previous work from a methodological point of view. Most previous work (and some since) has relied upon fixed choice questionnaires and interviews, (Lorber's work in 1975 is a good example) and thus has the fundamental weaknesses that actual behaviour towards patients is never examined, and that little of the context in which social judgement takes place is ever articulated. Kelly and May argue that much of the research fails to define concepts accurately enough for the positivistic analytic methods used to ensure validity and reliability.

Making a distinction between epistemological and theoretical criticism, Kelly and May nevertheless address in both sections their fundamental objections to what they term *neo behaviourism* and *reductionism* in previous research. By these they seem to mean that the research is simplistic and assumes that there are straightforward and predictable stimulus-response connections between variables which, once known, will cause nurses and others not to be judgemental about their clients. They suggest that much of the positivistic research has a 'high moral tone' implying that health workers and nurses in particular are in some sense wrong to hold negative views of their charges. They continue that whilst it may be wrong to do so, it is also inappropriate in dispassionate research endeavour to judge the attitudes and actions of research subjects without adequately observing and reporting upon wider contextual explanations of the noted behaviours and attitudes. As Kelly and May point out:

Scientific analysis of the processes involved (in defining patients as good and bad) may be perfectly permissible and desirable, but to have some idealised conceptions of a future more perfect system actually prejudges the issue and prejudices the research. (Kelly and May, 1982:152)

This criticism seems fair in relation to research which claims (at least implicitly) to be 'value-free', as much of the work using survey methods and quantification does (see also later work by Roberts, 1984). Where I would differ from Kelly and May would be to add the cautionary point that from a critical theory perspective such an alternative world can sometimes be clearly in mind, but the distinction is that in work using these perspectives such values and assumptions are more honestly stated (Punch, 1986; Webb, 1984).

Kelly and May's review is, because of space limitations no doubt, wide-ranging but does little to explore specific studies in any depth. Rather, they group studies by themes and methods and apply a broad critique which applies to most, but with exceptions. Nevertheless their study has much to commend it as an impetus to researchers in general, and nurses in particular, to investigate the use of naturalistic approaches (such as ethnography) in the study of social phenomena, such as social judgement.

As if to practise what they preach, these writers published a study of psychiatric nursing practice under the reverse authorship of May and Kelly, also in 1982. Drawing as they admit on data collected by observation and interview material 'rather fitfully collected over a period of four years' (p280), May and Kelly present what is in essence a case study of an individual psychiatric patient with some comparisons drawn with other patients. This highly naturalistic approach is, of course, consistent with their stated interactionist perspective and they seriously attempt to locate their theory of labelling of patients as problem patients in the social context in which the nurses they observed operate. In their introduction they argue that previous studies have ignored ambiguities and conflicts which are prevalent throughout nursing, but make a special case that a simplistic approach to the understanding of nurses' attitudes to patients is particularly inappropriate in psychiatric nursing. They imply that the principal source of conflict for nurses is the differing expectations that medical staff and patients have of nurses. This they argue is made worse because the authority of nurses in the mental health area is particularly fragile.

As is common in such reports, May and Kelly provide the usual disclaimer that their ideas are exploratory and not typical (or generalisable). Much of their rhetoric, however, betrays an opposite conclusion, that they speak of not only the two wards they studied but of all psychiatric nursing. An example is in their conclusion:

In this paper we have argued that problem patients for psychiatric nurses are those who in one way or another deny nurses' claims to therapeutic competence. (May and Kelly, 1982:295)

The possible weakness of their view stated above is its emphasis on psychiatric nurses. 'Problem' patients have been described in all types of clinical environment such as medical, surgical, rehabilitation and mental health, and care of the elderly (Fielding, 1986; English and Morse, 1988), and they themselves point this out at great length in their other paper (Kelly and May, 1982). May and Kelly seem to be at pains to separate out psychiatry as having unique features. These it may well have, but to isolate these as the necessary and sufficient cause of unpopularity and without addressing direct analytic comparison with other clinical contexts seems to reach beyond the data they provide.

I think that a plausible explanation of this is that as Kelly and May recognise in their other 1982 paper, unpopularity of patients with general nurses (of all types) cannot be explained by a traits approach of stereotyped behaviours and conditions. Despite this fundamental conclusion, in their own study they relapse into reliance upon traits research which refers to 'problem patients' in general nursing being possessors of certain qualities such as being 'pleasant and uncomplaining'. In examining a mental health setting they have concluded that something approaching a 'process' approach offers the best explanation of their findings, and have perhaps prematurely concluded that this applies only to psychiatric nursing.

Their analysis of the case of Doreen provides the basis of their theory that negative labels arise out of the patient's perceived responsibility for their actions and therefore their blameworthiness. Where the patient's actions challenge the nurses' right to use skill and knowledge in therapeutic endeavour, then the nurse will be frustrated at the challenge to an already fragile authority. Their power is said to be fragile because it is delegated by the doctor.

In relation to mental illness May and Kelly, despite referring to labelling theory in the ascription of mental illness and even the 'anti-psychiatry' movement, suggest that:

> ... all patients on a chronic psychiatric ward are presumably mentally ill, and therefore not, for the time being at least, responsible for their behaviour... (p288)

This rather simplistic assertion, assumes that a Parsonian (1951) sick role concept of illness behaviour is tenable in mental illness. That is to say that all persons once defined as ill by legitimate medical opinion are automatically exempted from responsibility for their behaviour. As Freidson (1970) points out:

> ... the individual's capacity is thought to be beyond the exercise of (his) own choice and so (he) is *not held responsible* for it. (p227, Freidson's emphasis)

This assumption, that such freedom from responsibility exists, has been much questioned by sociologists who have extended Parsons' analysis to account for the complexity provided by non-medical and non-acute illnesses. Freidson himself draws attention to the idea that illness, and especially mental illness, can most easily be seen as social state which persons assume rather than a necessarily objective and permanently recognisable biological state. May and Kelly then proceed to discuss degrees of blame and responsibility which patients were seen to have attached to them. Against the background of their apparent acceptance of

63

an overtly biological theory of mental illness their argument is hard to accept.

In summary, they claim that psychiatric nursing is different in a way which implies that their discussion has no relevance for other types of nursing. There is also some ambiguity in their allegiance to the labelling perspective in explaining the attribution of blame in mental illness. This is because when it is convenient to do so, they accept that medically constructed labels of mental illness are adequate to remove responsibility for actions from the individuals so labelled. Nevertheless, May and Kelly make a major advance upon all previous studies with perhaps the exception of Roth (1972) by noticing the importance of the nurse's power to define a person as a problem or otherwise, or in their terminology, *a chancer, a pest or a poor wee soul*. In particular they attempt to conceptualise social judgement as a flexible social process which is influenced by social and professional political factors and which is not necessarily a 'bad' thing to happen.

Another case history

Neil McKeganey's (1984) contribution offers even more detailed discussion of an individual case history which he acquired as a participant observer for four months in a therapeutic community in Scotland where children of varying degrees of developmental handicap were resident. McKeganey's paper is light on sociological theory and instead offers a very reflexive and detailed account of both his own and the staff's perceptions of the moral status of the particular individual highlighted. He draws attention early to the influence of May and Kelly in his interest in the phenomenon of moral evaluation of persons such as 'Linda', and is mainly concerned to illustrate how it is that the staff promulgate their perception of Linda as 'trouble' in order to manage or exert social control. That is to say the staff have their goals of care which Linda might easily frustrate unless she is labelled as 'trouble'.

McKeganey claims no more for his paper than ethnographic description and it is therefore difficult to criticise what might otherwise be seen as reluctance to set the study into the context of developed social theory that others have attempted (e.g. Dingwall and Murray, 1983).

Theoreticity and conventionality?

Dingwall and Murray's paper presents a substantial contrast to McKeganey's case study, drawing upon a minimum of observational data (seven four-hour sessions) mainly in one casualty department. Focusing on medical staff's categorisation of patients as good and bad, Dingwall and Murray (1983) outline the limitations of previous explanations of the labelling process (such as Jeffery, 1979) illustrating their argument by reference to children and their parents. They suggest that the categorisation of clients rests on the practical contingencies of the work (in this case emergency care), and on the social organisation of the work rather than a simple notion of the attenders at the department breaking 'rules' as both Jeffery (1979) and others have suggested. Dingwall and Murray show clearly how it is that children can break Jeffrey's' 'rules' and not be labelled bad (or 'rubbish'). By means of the example of children failing to fit any simplistic notion of social judgement of clients, they seem concerned to show that all 'rule-based' explanations of moral categorisation are potentially flawed.

On a reflexive note I will point out that their paper is at once valuable but complex. Dingwall often has the characteristic of addressing issues at a very high level of abstraction which seems in one sense dissonant with the otherwise naturalistic and open approach evident in his work. At risk of inadequately summarising their argument, I will nevertheless offer some initial comments upon the discussion he and Murray offer.

First they acknowledge the basic value of a simple notion of deviant rule-breaking in beginning a discussion of the moral evaluation (social judgement) of clients in a casualty department. They draw further attention to the rather obliquely named concepts of *theoreticity* and *conventionality* which are said to be qualities shown by an actor in performance of a potentially deviant act. Theoretic actors are those who can assess their action as being in or out of accord with some 'rule', the implication being that they can more easily be held responsible for such an act if they have the *theoretic* facility (because they knew they were transgressing). This idea can I think be conceptualised as *awareness*. Conventionality is behaviour which has been labelled by someone whose power to do so is socially recognised, as in breach of a rule where conformity to the rule would have been possible (Dingwall and Murray, 1983). Rephrased in 'older' sociological terms this latter concept, more easily grasped in its negative version as *unconventionality*, is the *primary deviance*. To summarise the way in which Dingwall and Murray extend Jeffrey's (1979) rather Parsonian analysis, I reproduce their table overleaf:

Table 2: Theoreticity and conventionality (after Dingwall
and Murray 1983 : 135)

	Conventional	**Non-conventional**
Theoretic	A. Breaks rules 　Responsible (appropriate patients)	B. Breaks rules Unavoidable Responsible (inappropriate Patients)
Pre-theoretic	B. Breaks rules 　Not responsible (Children)	D. Breaks rules Unavoidable Not responsible (Naive Patients)

Dingwall and Murray attempt to utilise this extension of the notion of the breaking of Jeffrey's (1979) four rules to show that not all persons who break the rules of therapeutic interaction are held responsible. Notably in their paper the focus is on children but also the 'naive' who might, I assume, be the semi or unconscious who are also 'pre-theoretic' and therefore are not supposed to attract blame.

Having spent some time coming to terms with the concepts of theoreticity and (non) conventionality, I can see something of the explanatory elegance which Dingwall and Murray apply as their test of other, in their view less adequate, formulations. I find however that my uncomfortable conclusion is that despite their assertion that simple rule-based explanations are weak, this account places its emphasis upon 'at least three classes of patients' (p134). It therefore places some considerable emphasis on traits of patients rather than processes. It also assumes a predictive power of a simplistic two times two table of categories which I would suggest is inconsistent with any concept of 'negotiation' of the categorisation or social evaluation arrived at.

Dingwall and Murray acknowledge in their final pages (p141) that "even 'bad' patients can become 'good' patients", and certainly locate their concluding argument more in terms of the social situation of junior doctors needing to get experience. Their thesis is that the special social status of children as 'precious' renders previously described clinical decision criteria for the award of a particular moral status to individuals irrelevant. Such a thesis therefore seems to me to imply also that other large categories of persons might defy the interpretation of their *moral status* in terms of such overarching classifications. Clearly claimed as an ethnography, primarily of one unit in terms of the observational data collected, the impression given is that all clinicians had the 'same' criteria for evaluation of 'rubbish' and that attitudes to clients were in some sense inevitable and universal. This is a claim which will bear further examination both in the medical and the nursing context.

Visiting attitudes

An Australian study published in a multi-national collection of monographs on communication was that by David Roberts (1984). He surveyed the degree of liking (using a Likert Scale) that 150 student nurses showed in relation to eleven specified categories of unpopular patients (identified from the literature). Examples included overdoses, aboriginal patients, terminally ill patients, psychiatric patients and patients with a drinking problem.

Some open-ended questions were asked and by these various means Roberts produces percentage frequencies of types of patients both liked and disliked. These naturally fall entirely into the traits approach except that he did ask nurses for some contextual information which is useful. 74% said that they had formed opinions about patients at handovers (change of shift reports). This finding, Roberts argues, lends support to bedside reports so that patients can be involved and objectivity will be increased.

Other data he reports which helps to change the orientation of the study from the determinism of the patients traits' approach are the opinions he sought upon why nurses changed their views of patients. 76% said they had indeed done this and gave reasons why. Some common reasons were given as 'time to talk with the patient', empathising with the patient, finding an underlying problem, realising the patient was lonely, and discovering the patient was in pain. Returning to cross-tabulations of biographical factors in the students which correlated with liking or disliking behaviour, Roberts reports a number of statistically significant findings such as that second year nurses liked caring for alcoholic patients. As is usual in such attitude surveys he can only speculate as to their importance. Roberts dismisses all observational techniques, arguing that:

Few of the (previous) researchers have addressed themselves to the inherent problems involved in conducting observational research in a ward setting. (Roberts, 1984:8)

Whilst quoting Olesen and Whittaker (1967), Jeanne Quint (1967) and of course Erving Goffman (all noted observers) in his general discussion,

67

Roberts fails to acknowledge their perspective or the relevance of their methods for this complex area of study.

Fielding's attitudes revisited

In 1985 Pauline Fielding reported the review of the literature (Ingham and Fielding, 1985) which formed the basis of her subsequent empirical study of nurses' attitudes to elderly patients (Fielding, 1986). In this selective and fairly critical examination of the preceding literature Fielding draws out the main emphases as:

1. characteristics of the nurses, such as age, sex, education;
2. characteristics of the patients, including behaviour and degree of institutionalisation;
3. effects of interventions such as educational programmes;
4. related nurses' attitudes such as willingness to work with older clients.

In summary Fielding attacks the majority of the work as follows:

> In general, aspects of the methodology of many of the studies are severely lacking, and in some cases the data presented are insufficient to allow adequate assessment. These factors not only make it difficult to compare studies against each other, but they also cast serious doubt on the reliability and validity, and hence the value, of the studies themselves. (Ingham and Fielding, 1985:178)

The severest attack is made upon quantitative attitude survey approaches which have been numerous in nursing research, and an example of which is the study by Roberts (1984) which is contemporary with Fielding's empirical work. Fielding (1986), in the main report of her work, argues that studies of attitudes which focus on simple behavioural or attitudinal items do not contribute to our understanding of the situations within which attitudes are expressed. She goes on to suggest that the approach she both used and recommends is rather superior in this respect. Working from an explicitly psychological perspective, Fielding argues that the collection of live interactions between nurses and their patients is the best way of inferring the attitudes which underlie them. To validate and contextualise the findings Fielding recommends an immediate *challenge* to the utterer to explain what they were saying and why, and in what context. This she attempted to do in three wards with student nurses as her 'subjects', reporting in some detail upon their conversations and their apparent meaning to the actors, in particular the students. Because

Fielding viewed unpopularity as a feature of being old she also asked the students how popular the patient they had been talking to was and why.

There is little doubt that the approach Fielding describes is essentially interpretive, with her as investigator being assisted in the collection of instances of nursing or other relevant phenomena by radio-microphones and tape recorders. She then explored ideas generated in informal interviews with participants. As she says herself this approach produced much rich data for analysis. Having gone to some lengths to disqualify deterministic 'trait' approaches in her review of other work however, it seems fair to suggest that she has not completely shaken off this tradition in her own analysis:

> The nature of the popularity of some of the patients in the present study is perhaps indicative of a need for further research in order to determine to what extent certain characteristics of patients may result in them being deprived of autonomy and independence.(Fielding, 1986:49)

Such a point shows that she still feels at the discussion stage of her analysis that it is patient traits which chiefly determine the outcome of their care. In other respects her claim that she has engaged in new methodological developments is fair in the wider context of a quantitative emphasis in most previous work.

Ethnography and 'ethnoscience'

Canadians Jennifer English and Janice Morse (1988) published an interesting paper about the 'difficult' elderly patient, which attempts a less haphazard methodological triangulation than Stockwell had done over a decade before. First, using what they call *ethnoscience*, they gathered data systematically from five qualified nurses. They began with tape-recorded unstructured interviews and moved on to card sort and sentence completion techniques to generate the nurses' perceptions and definitions of the types of patient that become difficult. This method, despite the arguably small sample for such a purpose, produced a wealth of rich descriptive data and a very wide taxonomy of potentially difficult behaviours which they show in a convenient table form.

Then using what they prefer to distinguish as *ethnographic techniques*, English and Morse interviewed and observed seven particular patients who had been perceived as 'difficult'. Making the not unreasonable claim that no previous authors had 'attempted to examine the phenomenon of 'difficult' from the patients' perspective' (p24), they identify a number of key factors or variables such as loss of control and power, lack of independence, lack of communication, lack of care, and lack of control of treatment. These they aggregate as the overarching category of *expectations not met*, the consequences of which are unpleasant emotions such as embarrassment and the consequent difficult behaviour. This *patients' model* has an elegance not found in much of the other research in that it is a conceptual framework with a process emphasis rather than a traits or individually focused one.

As a third part of the study, and to attempt to provide some predictive potential for the model, English and Morse reviewed an extensive but primarily prescriptive literature in the 'popular journals'. Their aim was to identify what methods had been considered successful in the management of difficult patients. Most of these papers were of the 'How to handle the crotchety, elderly patient' variety (Gasek, 1980) and so cannot form the basis of research-based practice. However as a review of nursing prescriptions which have been used and which warrant formal evaluation this part of the paper also has some limited merit. Since they have in some sense incorporated a wider literature of case studies into their model, English and Morse do seem to argue for a 'limited generalisability of findings' (p37) but they omit to say how limited. However they are keen to accept that the prescriptive elements of their model require validation in clinical settings.

In summary I believe that the authors are aware of the limitations and oversimplicity of the traits approach to understanding difficult or unpopular behaviour. Therefore they have attempted to contextualise their list of behaviours likely to predict unpopularity, with the addition of a patients' model which examines the importance of wider issues such as power and control.

Focusing on patients' perceptions

In a small qualitative study by Susan Waterworth and Karen Luker (1990) the focus is primarily upon whether patients really do want to be involved in decisions about their care. Interviewing twelve patients in total from three wards on a convenience and willingness basis, they noted the degree to which the patients had 'toeing the line' as a prime objective of their hospital stay. The relevance of this for my study, and as Waterworth and Luker suggest, is that patients comply with nurses' wishes in order to avoid unpopularity or 'getting into trouble'. They refer to Kelly and May's (1982) influential reminder that patients are not merely passive recipients of health care, but suggest that from their data patients were only too happy to hand over the responsibility for their welfare to the staff.

The paper offers an interesting hypothesis that, whilst current nursing curriculum ideology suggests that patients should be involved in decisions about their care, this does not seem to be what they want. Waterworth and Luker admit that their sample is small and do not refute the charge that patients they interviewed may have been 'toeing the line' in their interviews with the researcher(s) who are both experienced and senior nurses. By this I mean that it is hardly surprising to find that, those patients who when asked by a senior nurse to be interviewed willingly comply, use compliance as a major survival strategy in hospital. Despite these vulnerabilities this type of research is commendable because the investigators risk the problems and difficulties inherent in clinical research.

A later example of work which attempts to grasp the patients' perceptions of the health care experience in the context of negative social judgement is yet another of the studies of casualty departments. Helen Roberts (1992) continues in the tradition of Roth (1972), Jeffrey (1979) and Dingwall and Murray (1983) in trying to explain the social processes behind the use of casualty departments. As she points out, much of the relevant literature is about supposedly 'inappropriate' usage of this service. She argues that generally medical perspectives have implied abuse of the service by users who have complaints that could more 'appropriately' be dealt with elsewhere. Sociologists, she argues, have tended to act as apologists for clients in these circumstances, explaining attendance in terms of poor access to other services such as general practitioners. She further argues, in common again with Kelly and May (1982) (though not with explicit reference to them), that most accounts have tended to present patients (or parents) as passive recipients of health care rather than active caretakers of their own (or their children's) health.

Interviewing, in their own homes, parents who had recently attended a casualty department, Roberts presents both providers' and users' views of three key issues. These are being 'rubbish', 'being on the safe side', and 'resources'. In summary she concludes that whilst casualty services may well see themselves as specialist and 'for serious cases', the need for parents in particular to be on the safe side when their children present them with unusual illness behaviour overrides any consideration of unpopularity. In her introduction Roberts had suggested that sociologists had acted as apologists for patients, and in such terms it is hard to see how her thesis departs from a similar categorisation. She does however stress the active, and in many ways highly competent position which parents occupy in the negotiation of casualty services for their children. In comparison to the Dingwall and Murray (1983) paper she addresses theoretical issues to a far lesser degree, reporting data quite fully and in respondents' terms. She does however make comparisons between groups of respondents and draws theoretical inferences in her summaries. In one

71

other respect she offers a similar contribution however. In both papers there seems to be a moral message. This of course risks the accusation previously levelled mostly at the nursing literature by Kelly and May (1983) that there is a high moral tone. For Dingwall and Murray (1983) the message is 'take children seriously', and less explicit but equally present in Roberts work is the advice to take their parents seriously too.

Good and bad patients literature: summary and conclusions

I intend briefly to summarise my review of the literature on good and bad patients in three sections: first, methods used in this area of research; second, a note about theoretical perspectives or research traditions; and finally some key theories and concepts arising in what I believe to be influential work.

Methods

Many early studies both by nurses and other social and behavioural scientists were of the social survey type. Most were attitude surveys which attempted to discover variables, mostly in the patients, which were associated with popularity and unpopularity. Frequently, as with Lorber (1975) and Roberts (1984) there are conclusions which reach well beyond the foundations which survey approaches supply. Whilst drawing upon the work of important interpretive sociologists such as Goffman and Freidson for theoretical flavouring, data collection often owes more to convenience of computer analysis than a genuine attempt to explain social phenomena from the perspective of those involved. Kelly and May (1982) and to some extent Ingham and Fielding (1985) deserve recognition for their attempts to highlight these limitations from their respective sociological and psychological perspectives.

From my point of view those studies with most to offer in an understanding of the phenomenon of social judgement in the clinical social world are those in which data were collected in less structured ways. It seems to me that this tradition, which might loosely be termed the *Chicago School* (Denzin, 1992), has produced a good deal of powerful explanation and understanding of health care delivery, such as the influential work by Howard Becker (1961) and his associates. Julius Roth's (1972) paper is the first substantial effort in this area and with a specific focus on what he terms *moral evaluation*. His paper is the first contribution to use both naturalistic fieldwork or participant observation methods and to locate explanation beyond simplistic ideas of patients' behaviour, illnesses or attitudes.

I have discussed how it was that Stockwell's (1972) work made an advance in belatedly acknowledging the value of ethnographic description in attempting to salvage something worth having from an otherwise unsuccessful attempt to quantify variables predicting unpopularity. Among nurses, Fielding (1986) made a serious attempt to collect data from the clinical environment and to infer attitudes from behaviour rather than the clearly less successful (but rather more popular) other way around.

The most consistent efforts to generate a theory of social judgement or to modify it based upon observation of social actors in their social context have been made by British sociologists such as Strong (1980) and Dingwall and Murray (1983). Often using data rather sparingly in their discussions, they nevertheless write in relation to their lived experiences and those of their informants. Most importantly, they generally are consistent in their adoption of wider contextual explanations of the phenomena they discuss. Whilst they mostly use participant observation, this is clearly a form in which they remain sociologists. They are participants in a social setting (usually a Casualty department!) rather than playing the roles of nurses or other health workers. These insights are valuable, and it remains a source of concern that their methods and level of discourse are rarely emulated by nurses. Two of the many reasons for this would, I suggest, be the anxiety-provoking nature of clinical work of any kind and the greater expense in terms of hours and energy per unit of data collected.

Theories and important concepts

As I argue in the introduction to this section no theory marks a defined starting point to my study. Much nursing research has a pragmatic flavour and even in quantitative research where explicit theoretical frameworks might be expected they are often missing or poorly related to the aims and outcomes of the studies (see for example Lelean, 1973). However it is clear that, as with the voluminous literature on the sociology of professions and professionalism, there seem to be two broad orientations. The first, and still the most influential, is the traits theory. This carries with it the assumption that persons are evaluated as to their social worth in relation to one or more variables such as attitude, behaviour or medical diagnosis. Numerous studies operate with this assumption, such as that of Lorber (1975), and others are unable to escape its influence. Of these latter Fielding (1986) is the best example. Having done her best in other ways to describe the context of social judgement of patients by nurses, Fielding's discussion resumes a reductive traits approach:

It was apparent from the accounts that if not all patients were deemed to be outright popular, it was a minority who were judged to be overtly unpopular. In the main, these were the 'geriatric' patients in both units. (Fielding, 1986:49)

I suggest that, in common with the 'professionalism' literature, the competing theoretical orientation is one which emphasises social processes rather than individual traits. Investigators such as Roth (1972) and later British workers in this tradition such as Dingwall and Murray (1983) are clearly focused upon explanation of a negotiated order, one in which no simple set of variables predicts the evaluations professionals will make of their clients. Such attempts are naturally more allied to my own interpretive perspective but more work needs to be done in clarifying the assumptions held. Indeed Dingwall and Murray (1983) seem to spend a good deal of time modifying only slightly a Parsonian Functionalist analysis of social judgement in relation to rules derived from the sick role.

Process explanations seem to have ideas like power, control, attribution and negotiation in common. They share the assumption, which Kelly and May (1982) and others articulate forcefully, that patients or their advocates often play a vital and far from passive role in the social judgement of persons as it occurs in health care contexts. Of nursing research reviewed, only the small study by English and Morse (1988) makes a serious attempt to construct a model which takes account of the perceptions of clients, and which does not wholly lose sight of a process orientation. I therefore remain assured that further contributions using naturalistic approaches to develop what is a very weak theoretical base are not misplaced.

6 Judging people and assessing

Judging people

In this chapter I aim to describe the phenomenon of social judgement with reference to examples from my fieldwork. As they arise, I will introduce relevant theoretical issues and research to illustrate further (or to contradict) ideas which arise from the data. I will present evidence that people in hospital are sometimes labelled postively or negatively. More than this, I will begin to show how the process is complex in a way not previously appreciated in the literature. That is, it is flexible, negotiable, impermanent and impossible to predict according to straightforward criteria or traits. I will illustrate the role of first impressions, in *assessing*, but will make clear that stereotypes have only a moderate and impermanent effect upon social reputation.

I had been on the ward undertaking my 'real' fieldwork for only one whole day when a particular idea became inescapable. I had known that my agenda was fairly open, indeed I was really hoping that I would be in some way describing how nurses made moral decisions or something of that kind. In fact I was doing my best to focus on situations where the nurses were faced with difficult moral choices to allow something like this to crystallise. It soon became clear that people in the ward were commonly discussed in terms other than the purely functional or 'professional'. On my second day I made a note in my book as follows:

Some patients are distinctly popular and some unpopular. This does not easily fit them as stereotypes however. Neil (a 23 year old with complications of a sexually transmitted disease) has an arguably stigmatising illness, and (being rendered very immobile from arthritis) is very demanding in the sense of knowing what he wants. He seems very popular however. He says "thank you" after everything.

75

Other entries in my field diary confirm these impressions. "He's a good lad" and "a nice patient" were two other opinions of Neil given to me within hours by different qualified nurses.

It would be unfair of me to argue that this notion of popularity or its opposite is original, far from it. Indeed I was sensitive to the idea both from my own practice and from the influential work of others. Felicity Stockwell's (1972) study *The Unpopular Patient* probably ranks among the most quoted studies of British Nursing. I myself had been impressed by Kelly and May's (1982) comprehensive review and critique of the relevant literature surrounding the topic of *Good and Bad Patients*. I had perhaps seen their paper too much as a convenient list of factors which promote or inhibit popularity, and had even used it thus in my teaching. Being aware of the issue, I thought that an open agenda approach to data collection would lead me to select instances of moral difficulty of some other type. To pursue the popularity question vigorously would mean me testing hypotheses rather than generating new ones.

However, I was struck by the importance of the issue and began to realise that, whatever the problems it raised, I would have to explore the idea further. I would just resolve to be open about the degree to which my notions of good and bad patients were pre-conceived. I decided to avoid re-reading the Kelly and May paper until my data base was more substantial, although I need not have been so worried. The paper, whose concluding argument I had perhaps not fully grasped in 1982, makes a strong case for a fresh examination of the good and bad patients issue from an interactionist perspective in which naturalistic qualitative methods would inevitably play a major part.

"He's charismatic"

Neil Tomlinson, the 23 year old young man suffering severe Reiter's Syndrome arthritis had much to endear him to nursing staff. He was polite, thanked the nurses after they had helped him, and was roughly the same age as the qualified nurses and many of the students. Some clearly felt pity for his situation, describing it as "very sad" although I did not know the whole story at this point. Somehow it was easy to see Neil fitting the traditional criteria for likability, similarity of age and politeness being examples. Popularity as a patient was not confined to Neil however.

Douglas (Doug) Whitbread was popular too, but it was hard to see why. This elderly man was likely, by any commonsense notion of patient popularity, to be seen in a very poor light. The research literature would confirm these suspicions. He was old, aged 82, which by itself risks unpopularity on an acute medical ward, with the patient being perceived as 'in the wrong place' or 'taking up an acute bed' (Baker, 1978). Douglas was suffering from chronic congestive cardiac failure and chronic bronchitis. These diagnoses were common on the ward, but he was unusual. Whilst the medical staff prescribed aggressive medication (such as a diuretic injection by intravenous pump) and a severe (500mls) fluid (drinks) restriction, he failed to comply with this regime in all its important respects. He would drink copiously from a hidden Fanta (orangeade) bottle, and would regularly empty his bladder into the toilet so that his urine volume could not be recorded.

Many studies suggest that deviant or rule breaking behaviour results in staff perceiving patients as bad (Armitage 1980, Habenstein and Christ, 1963). Kelly and May (1982) refer to eleven papers which suggest that patients who persistently fail to conform to the clinical regime "will be regarded unfavourably". Douglas smoked very heavily indeed. He smoked roll-ups virtually constantly and spent almost all of every day and night in the day room in which he and others were allowed to smoke. This behaviour was clearly contra-indicated in his condition, and was the more anti-social for being partly the source of Doug's unkempt and often dirty appearance. He was covered in cigarette ash and both he and his clothing had an inevitably strong nicotine smell. He regularly refused to bathe or be bathed, and this factor too, would, according to many studies, lead him to be negatively evaluated by staff (Kelly and May,1982).

Some research (Altschul, 1972) suggests that social class differences can contribute to negative social evaluation of patients. Douglas had been a tram and bus driver for over forty years, and whilst some of the nurses undoubtedly had working class origins, their education, role and function as nurses in a large City Teaching Hospital had inevitably increased the social distance between them and him.

But Doug was popular! When I began to explore his popularity with Helen, a second year student nurse, she had her own theory:

MJ: Would you say Doug Whitbread was popular or unpopular?

Helen: Popular! ... But he's not very demanding is he?

MJ: No.

Helen: He can be,...but he's sort of charismatic.

MJ: He breaks the rules, he doesn't comply with treatment at all, he drinks Fanta out of a bottle and smokes roll-ups, and yet you're right, he's got something that overrides the other factors that should make him unpopular... It's not a simple thing at all.

Helen: Then you can't defend why you like someone and why you don't outside the job, so... I still think there's too much favouritism and its expressed too openly. You'll hear it in report: "I really like him", which says a lot.

"He's a lovely man"

Being seen as a good patient was not at all unique. Quite commonly, some evaluative comment was added to the other factual nursing and medical information flow, particularly during ward reports. One patient, awaiting transfer to another ward for extensive heart surgery, was introduced to me with "he's a lovely man". Mr. Patel was of Asian origin but had been in the United Kingdom for thirty years, and had exceptional command of English. He was quiet, compliant, and seemed on the face of it to be relatively unperturbed by his impending open heart surgery.

He was mobile and in all physical respects self-caring. I made a point of doing his observations and talking to him to try to find out why he was 'lovely'. He was quiet, completely unquestioning of our interventions and those suggested by the medical staff. But the label helped me interact with him with less fear of him being awkward or hard to converse with, whatever stereotypical impression I may have had of Asian bus drivers before. The label 'lovely' helped to overcome any fear of the potential culture gap. I knew that the interaction would be a safe one and that embarrassment arising out of our dissonant cultural and ethnic backgrounds would be at a minimum.

Sometimes good patient labels were applied in a very ambiguous way, one in which differing opinions were expressed in the same breath or at the same time. One example of this was Jimmy MacKindoe, a Glaswegian who had, despite spending most of his adult life in England, never lost his regional Scottish accent. Jimmy had had a stroke, and being rather disabled was consequently quite dependent for some weeks. As he later began to improve quite remarkably, it was discovered he also had a malignant tumour of the lung, which was inoperable. Jimmy did not know this latter diagnosis, and seemed when I met him to be trying very hard to develop enough mobility to be accepted in an old people's home. Somehow, the personal evaluations of Jimmy were ambiguous in a way which my conversation with third year student nurse Olivia crystallised very well:

Olivia: ...I find him quite...I'm jumping the gun here... I mean he's a great bloke, he is attention-seeking, again who isn't? Losing half your body is a horrible thing to happen to you, and I think he's played a blinder to be quite honest. You should have seen him five weeks ago...everybody seems to have quite a negative attitude to him because, I don't know why, usually if someone was like that and they were getting over a stroke, and they found out they (patient) had cancer, they'd be absolutely mortified. If it was anyone else they'd be really upset. But I don't know what it is about him that nobody gives a monkey's really.

Olivia seemed to convey the ambivalence and the guilt that the nurses felt about labelling Jimmy in the way that they did. They seemed to be identifying the reasons why they should like him, and then admitting to and trying to explain the fact that they did not. This complexity is hard to understand in terms of straightforward criteria of likability an unpopularity, and is extended by the notion of covert liking which seemed to exist.

Covert liking

Some nurses felt disposed to stress to me both in my informal discussions with them and in the formal interviews that they somehow liked patients when no-one else seemed to:

MJ: I'm trying to work out what the distinction is: what the popular ones are doing right and the unpopular ones doing wrong. what do you think is the difference?

Helen: I do find it very strange becasue we have a very casual report, so these things come across, and while I don't want the report to be normal, there is too much favouritism. A gentleman on his ward a few weeks ago, everybody hated him, personally I found him very appealing because he reminded me of my father, and that did upset me to hear them talking about him like they did.

This conception of liking was common, but had an 'off the record' quality. By this I mean that it was implied that I could use the idea, but that I must protect anonymity scrupuloulsy in doing so. Among others, a second year student Theresa summed up the risks attached to liking people whom others did not:

Theresa: ...I feel sorry for the people who feel unpopular and no-one likes them and we (nurses) often feel reluctant to come out in the open and say "I like this or that person". I just keep my head down really.

I will develop this idea more fully in examining the strategies used by the nurses in manageing care by using evaluative labels generally. I have alluded to some of the properties of liking such as ambiguity and secrecy. Indeed such complexity contradicts a simplistic picture of 'popularity'.

79

Another dimension of liking was its changability over time and under differing conditions. Discussing the factors which promoted likability, Louise pointed this out to me also noting the need to keep dissident views to oneself:

Louise: ...And then I've noticed that the attitude has changed on occasion, not because the patient's behaviour changed, but because their condition may have worsened, the attitude toward them may change..

MJ: Suddenly people feel kindlier toward them?

Louise: Yeah! I think it's a shame because, like I say, I don't feel on this ward now, that I...I've spoken up on occasions and don't feel that it's been accepted, and it's been very hard to sit there and stand up for what you think has been said that shouldn't have been said. You know people might be put down.

Being unpopular

My early field work was suggesting that evaluative labels were an important way of managing interpersonal relations. Both my fieldnotes and the interviews were conveying the distinct impression that, although some labels were positive, those about which my informants felt most strongly were of a different sort. Nurses at all levels of experience knew precisely what I meant when I asked about popularity and unpopularity. Their responses at interview were immediate and as if I had, in each case, touched a nerve. They wanted to tell me about their experiences and my sense of the immediacy of the issue to these informants increased with each successive interview:

Helen: ...and I don't mind what goes on in, like, small interactions but, especially when you've been introduced to a patient and you're told that "they're miserable"...

MJ: They're labelled?

Helen: Yeah!

Helen's view was confirmed by the much more experienced third year nurse Olivia:

MJ: You seem to be saying that some patients, Jimmy (McKindoe) in particular, are less popular than others.

Olivia: Yeah, I mean he does ask for things if you pass him but he goes out of his way now to say "If you don't mind, I won't take long" and all this. It's shocking really...how just one person

80

	can colour everybody's opinion. It's happened a lot in the case of Jimmy. He's not a bad bloke, and he really does try, unlike a lot of people. He doesn't need a kick up the arse at all.
MJ:	So you think that the kind of informal labelling that goes on is quite powerful really?
Olivia:	Yeah, I think I do it as much as everyone else really.

Olivia brough the issue into the discussion unprompted, and was clearly concerned about its potential effects. Yet she had a lively appreciation of her own role in labelling and was commenting upon the lack of a simple explanation for it. Interviewing my next respondent I mentioned it quite early on in our discussion:

MJ:	Do you think that some of the patients are unpopular?
Bill:	Yeah! without a doubt! I've never seen it affect nursing care as such, maybe on a personal cleanliness level it hasn't, but on a psychological level it does because they (nurses) don't spend as much time with the patient or find time to chat. They just want to get the job over and done with in a way, and then move on...

Bill was a most insightful respondent, despite being at the end of only his first ward allocation when interviewed. I was worried about the leading nature of the question when I was waiting for the response, but its coherence in differentiating between the physical and psychological consequences of negative labels reassured me that Bill was giving me his own perceptions and not just what I wanted to hear. Whenever I asked about unpopularity the reply was definite. Yes it exists and yes, it is a problem. My data began to yield a large number of examples of labels with which nursing staff communicated their negative social evaluations of the people in their care. I intend now to proceed with a description of some of these before examining the conditions under which labels seem to be used and the purposes they may serve.

Being demanding: "oh, he's a right one!"

I began to explore the nature, or the properties of these negative labels, so that I could formulate some notion of their place in managing care on the ward.

Bill:	...I mean, I was surprised myself really coming to the wards, you know, hearing people literally slagged off, and it seemed really strange to me at first, but you get used to it.

Bill's experience was not untypical. He had anticipated that there would be fewer personal evaluations used in discussing patients, but had begun to accept this norm. I could not help noticing however in working with the students, that (first ward student) Bill was widely perceived as able to disregard the normative opinion of a patient, and give them as much attention as he felt appropriate. Indeed one of my third year informants was keen to point this out:

Olivia: You know, people in the office (qualified nurses) were saying "Jimmy Mackindoe's getting far too demanding" and Bill didn't discriminate, he had time for him. And I thought "that's good, you haven't coloured his opinion".

Olivia, with three years' experience of differing ward cultures, was aware of the process of negative labelling and its potential to affect the quality and amount of care. Being 'far too demanding' seems at first like a condition under which a negative attitude might arise. Being demanding did, however, convey a meaning beyond this. Demanding can mean challenging but not necessarily unpleasant, such as a difficult game or sport. It can also mean asking for that which is due, but in a fairly aggressive manner. Observation gave me the impression that being demanding was a descriptive label not necessarily related to the holder's propensity to ask for things. It was subtly different. Being demanding was a term used to convey dislike, although it often did apply to those who knew what they wanted and made a point of telling us. It conveyed not merely the fact that an individual was likely to make their expectations of the nurse very clear, it meant that they would do more than this. They were likely to 'overdo it'. An example from my field notes may illustrate this:

Charles Eastwood is fairly unpopular! He's 60(ish), has severe pneumonia and chronic airways disease. He's very "demanding" (word used in ward report) and the nurses are easily irritated by him. He leaves sputum-ridden tissues lying all over (which stick to you when you attempt to turn him) and has no humility at all in telling nurses where and how to wipe his bottom (he leaks constantly due to chronic constipation). He is clearly very ill and I'm doing my best to keep an open mind with him...

This field note reveals my assumptions about how people should ask to have their bottoms wiped! I imply in my hastily written note that he should have been more humble. On reflection I cannot justify this assumption except by appealing to current social conventions. Indeed this sort of incident sensitised me to the interplay between my own need to evaluate and label people and their behaviour, and my discovery of this tendency in others. However, my feelings about it were not untypical, and so the sense in which Charles was 'overdoing it', at least as far as nurses were concerned, is evident.

It is interesting that this quite special use of the word *demanding* stands up to international comparison rather well. Wolf (1988) undertook an ethnography of a medical ward in a large urban hospital in the United States of America using participant observation. She describes nurses routinely complaining about their patients in change of shift reports as follows:

> Most of these patients were labelled "demanding". Jenny Fister, an elderly patient with advanced heart disease, was dying slowly. Known as a demanding or complaining patient, she engendered anger and frustration in the nurses who cared for her. Mrs. Fister had been a patient on 7H for over a month; her outlook was grim and her nursing care a challenge. She never claimed to feel better. Her nurses felt encouraged that what they did for Mrs. Fister made a difference. Although they cared for Mrs. Fister daily, she never acknowledged their care. (Wolf, 1988, p.257)

I think that this use of the word demanding reflects very accurately that emerging from my fieldwork. It is a pejorative rather than merely a functional label. Bill, the first ward nurse was something of a key informant in the early part of my fieldwork, and provided me with much to think about. He indicated the way in which some labels are almost permanent, and can be based upon previous opinions of an individual:

Bill: ...Some of the patients have been in time and time again, so when you first come they say "Oh, he's a right one him" and when you see for yourself you think "he's not that bad really", but you've still got this preconceived idea of what he's like. You can't make your own judgement sometimes.

This suggests that labels are sometimes carried for long periods, and can be re-introduced when patients are re-admitted. Some labels used a terminology much less genteel than "he's a right one" or "he's demanding", but this depended very much upon the nurse using it. Conventional wisdom has it that in their professional context nurses use relatively polite language. I had found personally that in the majority of settings this was the case. Only once in my career, working in an intensive care unit, had I been surprised by colleagues of both sexes using strong or barrack room language to describe their patients. This sort of language was not very common, and certainly was uttered with the aim of being out of earshot of patients in particular, and also those nurses perceived to be of more delicate constitution. Olivia, the third year student who was both witty and particularly pragmatic, would use these terms in a way that, knowing her, you knew they were not worse than other pejorative terms. At coffee time one day Olivia bemoaned her dealings with an ill but recovering patient with severe alcoholic liver disease. "That Robert Munro really gets up my arse" was her honest appraisal of her feelings after a particularly trying few minutes talking to him. Now, at coffee time she felt at liberty to unload this view to me and the other student nurses present. Olivia had a directness of speech which out of context would have seemed coarse, but at the time seemed appropriate, if unorthodox.

One of the staff nurses also used this type of language, referring to one patient as "an old bastard". The use of such language carried a high degree of risk both for the user and, it seems to me, for those about whom it was used. It could be seen to break norms of professional conduct. Out of context, for example as evidence in a disciplinary hearing, such language about patients would be hard to justify. The risk to patients that the attitude of other nurses would harden toward them was always present. But although such labels were sometimes used, in context and with knowledge of the behaviour and commitment of the nurse using them, it was hard to discover any greater degree of malevolence in these labels than others such as "he's a right one" or "demanding".

The discussion of unpopular labels so far has focussed upon some types of relatively permanent labels. Others had a more transient nature, seeming to be used to deal with specific events or moods the patient might be perceived to be in. "He's really grumpy today" was an example of a label used about an elderly patient with an untreatable malignant tumour whom many nurses liked, because he was stoical and needed relatively little attention. On the day in question, however, he had been talked into a colonoscopy and gastroscopy to investigate loss of blood (examination of bowel and stomach by tube passed into the relevant orifices). He was undertaking strong laxative treatment to "clear his passages" and being already ill was not in the best of moods. This patient, Jack Redford, recovered from these investigations. Later, however, he wanted to go home, seeing little point in further investigations, and made his view known very clearly. This led to him being categorised as "in a real strop today".

"He's in a right strop" was also a label used to describe the mood of Robert Munro, the Scot who had been admitted to recover from tuberculosis and alcoholism. Robert was constantly the recipient of permanent labels, but when particularly difficult to deal with nurses would warn each other with an extra pointer. One such time was when doctors tried to take Robert off his sedative medication (chlormethiazole and chlordiazepoxide), drugs upon which he had come to rely very heavily. He became very angry and asked to complain to senior administrative staff. These extra and more temporary labels were generally reserved for the nursing team, but occasionally junior medical staff would be granted access to one. On this day, when Robert had asked to see a doctor to justify his complaint, the staff nurse suggested to the unsuspecting physician, "Take a crucifix with you".

"It's getting worse"

Labels can change. Catherine was a staff nurse with a quiet and thoughtful temperament. She seemed patient and unlikely to respond inappropriately to provocation. Furthermore she had considerable ability to articulate her insight into the moral dilemma of labelling. During my fieldwork we had conversations about a number of issues, and she seemed very ready to be more formally interviewed with the tape recorder:

MJ: Do you think some of the patients are unpopular?
Catherine: Definitely...It's on the verge of becoming a problem actually, because he (Albert Littlewood) has been in hospital for now, over a week, and it's getting a lot worse and he's getting a lot worse. I don't know if he's feeling a lot of antagonism, I mean I know I've got a lot of antagonism and find him hard to deal with, and I think I'm fairly tolerant, I don't get riled that easily.

Catherine seemed to be saying that a person's popularity can change over time, so I asked her to clarify this for me:

Catherine: I think it's easier to be unpopular and become popular. I think at first Albert Littlewood wasn't unpopular at all.
MJ: No?
Catherine: And it's just got worse, and it's getting into quite a bad situation. I can't remember when it was like this. It makes you think, "well if I'm a professional I'm not reacting in a professional way because I'm letting my feelings affect my behaviour".

Catherine felt the dilemma acutely, even more because she saw herself as a role model for students, and felt that she was letting down both patients and students in betraying her feelings about this patient. She seemed to use the notion of professionalism to mean being in control, not letting her personal feelings affect the care she gave. The consequences of labelling then, can be deeply felt, a feature I will aim to explore later.

Judgemental social evaluations of ward inmates, then, were common. Some were temporary and in some cases labels became relatively permanent. Some labels were subject to change over time. It seemed to me that Charles Eastwood became more liked as his condition improved and he became more independent. At this time he became easier to talk to, and I found that we had a number of common interests. A similar situation applied to Doug Whitbread, the elderly man with heart failure who according to the staff was failing to comply with most of his treatment. As he became less breathless it became possible to talk without exhausting him, and he suddenly became a person. In a note I taped after a day on the ward I made the observation that "I'm beginning to warm to him now". This was as a result of a long conversation in which he showed me a range of old photographs which explained much of his early life (he was 82). I could not help identifying with him though, when it became obvious he had known my father who worked at the same bus and tram depot. They had shared most of their working lives.

"He's weeing in the sink"

It is important to recognise that social judgement is not the sole province of the staff, patients also label each other. Throughout my fieldwork I was aware of an undercurrent of comment by patients in the ward about each other. My own experiences in the role of relative or visitor had sensitised me to the notion of ward inmates quite rapidly constructing opinions about the medical condition and likely prognoses of other patients.

The day room, being often smoke-filled, was rarely frequented by nurses. We would venture in to do a blood pressure or return a patient to his bed, but for much of the time this area was one in which patients could discuss staff or each other in relative privacy. It was my impression that I had access to much that nurses said that was 'off-stage', but this was not generally true of the men in the ward. However, I did obtain some little insight into the evaluative labelling which patients were involved in.

One day, John McGee (an elderly man with arthritis of his knees) drew my attention to another patient of similar age at the opposite end of his bay. "He's trying to wee in the ward sink" was Mr. McGee's accusation about this other man. He went on to say how this behaviour clearly showed what an "unhygienic and antisocial" person this other man, Albert Littlewood, was. Mr. McGee told me how he felt it was his responsibility to inform me as a member of the nursing staff, so that I could do something about the matter. It was clear that the complainant was indeed disgusted and expected me to account at a later point for the action I had taken. I agreed I would see what was actually happening and do my best to reduce any cause for embarrassment.

Later that afternoon Albert Littlewood was standing by the ward sink, with his trousers round his ankles, in full view of his accuser and anyone else who might have walked past. On close examination, however, he was actually trying to use a urine bottle, and was running the taps at the sink to attempt to assist his urine to flow. It was clear that Albert Littlewood was not liked by his colleague and that, whatever his behaviour, it was being interpreted as inappropriate at best and more likely as disgusting. The actual accusation of urination into the sink was unjustified but it served to focus attention upon an approach to excretion that was too public for Mr. McGee's taste.

Being "dirty" was a label applied by the young Neil Tomlinson to the elderly Jack Redford one day when Neil was chatting to student nurses at the nurses' station. Known for his politeness, Neil seemed genuinely upset by the low level of Jack's general cleanliness, and the fact that he swore much of the time. Neil seemed to be arguing to have Jack's bed moved to a different part of the ward, but if he was, he did not achieve his aim. Part of the reason the bed was where it was, was that Jack needed easy access to the toilets as he was having purgatives as preparation for endoscopies.

Neil and John McGee's readiness to complain about their inmate colleagues to nurses, seemed to be because of their view that these patients were breaking norms of cleanliness, particularly in toilet related behaviour. The importance as a property of evaluative labels was that the origin of these negative evaluations was fellow patient inmates.

Assessing: beginning social judgement

Here I will aim to develop the notion of judging people by illustrating the role of people in general and nurses in particular in constructing the labels which apply to persons in the ward. This phenomenon, as the beginning of a process of social judgement in Howarth ward can be termed assessing. This I think conveys the sense in which the process of labelling and the process of assessing patients' clinical and other capabilities are intertwined. I will now focus upon the role and influence of nurses in the social construction of patient identity. Inevitably the main actors under discussion are nursing staff, but some light may be shed upon the limited but important part that patients have to play in the social influence processes.

"You're only human"

My staff nurse informant, Neil, was always very keen to keep me in touch with the issues as he perceived them, and was very open about some of his feelings. I was impressed by his honesty in admitting quite easily that liking everyone was unrealistic, and that we all bring with us prejudices and irritations that it is hard to ignore:

Neil: I think patients can be unpopular for a number of reasons and not just being "moaners". I think that, for whatever reason, you just don't like the patient, and then from your point of view that patient is not number one in the popularity stakes.

On another occasion in a relatively informal chat, a staff nurse told me how they had a natural revulsion to an individual with a particular congenital deformity. The staff nurse said: "I know it's wrong," but it "couldn't be helped." This disclosure made me uneasy, but I couldn't tell why. I considered that on the one hand the staff nurse was being honest and informative, since I believe they understood very well what my research role meant. On the other I was aware of the 'observer effect' that I might be having. Some nurses took this role of 'honest commentators' whenever I seemed interested, and over the whole period of fieldwork I gained many insights from nurses who became key informants.

Third year student Olivia, also something of a key informant, agreed that whilst it was unrealistic to be able to get on with everyone, it was even less so to keep these opinions private:

Olivia: I don't think you can help it because you're only human. If someone's getting on your nerves there's no point in not admitting it, that's even falser.

These nurses clearly espoused a sort of realism, an appreciation that it was inevitable that people will have likes and dislikes, and that at least among peers it would be alright to mention them. Other nurses were worried by it, however. Elaine, who felt that it might be necessary to discuss opinions of patients with other qualified nurses, was clearly concerned that as a role model for student nurses she should avoid judging or pre-judging patients in this way:

Elaine: It's personal really, you can have personal differences, and that can make an unpopular patient. If they've got a personality that you don't 'gel' to. But I don't think you should voice them. Other than like qualified members of staff, I don't think students should ever be there when someone...but it's difficult when someone gets on your nerves very much.

Clearly Elaine's ideal would be to avoid labelling patients negatively or perhaps positively when students are around. Catherine, among others echoed similar views, and guilt that on one notable occasion and in the presence of students she had been particularly disparaging about Albert Littlewood. She too seemed to see no alternative to *segmenting* her behaviour, whenever she had the emotional resources, so that students would not be exposed to what she felt was a negative role model. Melia (1987:161) utilises the concept of segmentation to explain the different ways in which student nurses behave in order to 'it in' with two very different areas of their work, the College and the ward. It seems that some of the qualified nurses also have this sort of conception of the ideal or professional way of working, and the real or ward way. For some of the qualified nurses this segmentation is between two general ways of communicating. One, which is realistic and 'only human', is that in which they betray their perceptions of patients as good and bad. The alternative, of communicating only 'objectively' they see as morally and therefore educationally superior since they are employed at least partly as role models for student nurses. That they cannot achieve this ideal seems to lead to guilt or moral dissonance.

Staff nurses, then, were conscious of their responsibility, in lieu of their formal status, to behave professionally, that is in accordance with the ideal. Students, were also aware of the power of some individuals to initiate and then promulgate a particular view of someone. Third year student Anita suggested that certain members of staff had special powers to define the ward view of patients, and sometimes other people such as nurses and doctors:

MJ: What do you think it is that gets people labelled as unpopular?

Anita: It tends to come from a dominant personality amongst the staff. Expressing a sort of dislike of somebody,and then that tends to get picked up by others, personally I tend to like the ones people don't like.

Anita certainly felt that one or more dominant figures on the staff had special authority to cause labels to stick. She, along with many others, also felt that whilst she might privately disagree, she would normally be unable to challenge this dominant orientation. I had my hunches about which of the nurses had this power, but Anita was reluctant to confirm them herself, and I was reluctant to ask. I could not help feeling that

89

Anita had felt alienated from qualified groups of staff, that is she perceived her 'differentness' and lower status very acutely indeed. She told me about an occasion when she had felt very upset when a patient in another setting had asked for help, and the qualified staff had told her that he was just manipulating her:

Anita: I felt angry with the staff, the whole 'professional' atmosphere, that hadn't actually responded to that man's need.

She used the word professional, as far as I could tell from her inflection, in a sarcastic way, one in which she implicitly questioned the patient-centredness of the staff on that particular other unit. Anita, then, felt that individuals with dominant personalities, and perhaps formal status, could set the values of the group, and further, that dissidence was very difficult to sustain in the role and position of student.

Medical staff

The nurses were not the only source of social judgements of people on the ward. They were, as I have pointed out, the people whose culture I was most able to observe and participate in. I have also argued that high status, whether formally or informally ascribed, gave power to create and perpetuate a good or a bad label. In this context it would be wrong to omit mention of medical staff, even though they and their social processes were not the focus of my study. I had fairly limited contact with medical staff. Many of the nursing staff also saw relatively little of medical staff on their visits to the ward, which amounted to only fairly short periods of the day in most cases, during which they would relate mostly to the senior ward nurse only. I did, however, gain one or two fascinating insights into the categorisation of people by medical staff upon other than purely diagnostic criteria.

On one occasion, a senior registrar undertook a ward round of the sort which was really aimed at preparing her and her colleagues for the visit of the consultant for a more formal ward round of the patients the following day. She was accompanied by two other doctors, the house officer (HO) and a senior house officer (SHO). As the staff nurse in charge was busy, she asked me to accompany these doctors as she would have any of her more experienced colleagues. I knew the patients, so I felt happy to do this. I was also more able to write things in my notebook fairly openly as this behaviour is the norm when listening to the statements made by physicians during their ward rounds. I introduced myself to the senior registrar, whom I recognised from years previously, and who I think recognised my face as one she had met in the past, but without really knowing where and when. My field notes are revealing:

> (After seeing two or three patients) on his way down the ward, the SHO makes light of his uncertainty about some of the patients' histories. "We've got some pretty poor historians here" he says.

At the time I realised that this was medical jargon for someone from whom it was hard to get accurate information, the assumption being that they were not very bright. We were about to visit a Ronald Dyson, who had been admitted with apparent chest pain and had been transferred to the ward from the coronary care unit:

> As we approach Mr. Dyson, the senior registrar says, "Shall I shoot myself in the head before I get there?" (She has not met this man before). Both doctors smile.

Dr. Gray, the senior registrar has clearly gained the impression from her colleague, before even meeting this individual, that he will be rather stupid, and that interviewing him for a medical history will be onerous. Instead, they choose to see the whole anticipated interaction as a source of fun. My fieldnotes continue with a record of how, in the light of this situation their suspicions are confirmed, and Mr. Dyson does seem 'thick' by their criteria:

> The SHO confirms: "He has a large enzyme rise" (meaning that he has probably had a myocardial infarction), but when asked about when he last had pain he (Mr. Dyson) says "Sunday". Today is now Monday, so that this remark conflicts with an earlier statement Mr. Dyson made that he had not had pain now "for ages". When pressed Mr. Dyson agrees that he has had no pain since admission. This of course confirms the doctors' suspicions about his lack of clarity and he looks "thick" to them. "I see what you mean", says Dr. Gray, the senior registrar as they move away.

The medical staff, then, were quite likely to use first impressions and informal evaluations of patients' personal qualities in their professional judgements. In this case there was an objective ring, that is to say the judgement was supposedly base upon the frustration experienced by doctors when patients are poor historians. What was especially interesting was that this whole interchange took place on the ward, in transit between two patients' beds, and probably within the earshot of any listener. The retreat into the jargon of 'poor historian' was perhaps meant to keep lay persons such as other patients in ignorance of the meaning of the label, which to me was without doubt on this occasion.

Discussion: the concepts of social judgement and assessing

Moral questions in general, and social judgement (or moral evaluation) in particular have been widely discussed in a large number of works of various kinds in the humanities and in the social and behavioural sciences (Roth, 1972; English and Morse, 1988).

I have referred to the not inconsiderable attention the phenomenon has attracted in studies of the provision of health services, as reviewed by Kelly and May (1982) and others. However, during my work as a participant observer at City General Hospital, the concept assumed an importance I could not ignore. Although untrained in the skills and methods of philosophy, my overwhelming area of interest was moral questions. I had therefore decided to attempt to inform debate about such moral questions by improving the empirical basis of such discussions (insofar as my study would allow).

My sensitivities, which I freely admit, were to moral questions such as the (perhaps) unjustifiably aggressive pursuit of treatment and the infliction of discomfort and pain, among many such important issues. It was soon very clear to me that I would be wrong to ignore what I now call social judgement on the ward. As my data make clear, the expression of evaluations of social worth was widespread on the ward, whether in terms of 'good and bad patients' (Kelly and May, 1982) or 'popular and unpopular' ones (Stockwell, 1972).

My argument, for which I believe I provide empirical and theoretical support in this book, is that social evaluations are not in any clear way tied to traits or variables which patients do or do not possess. Rather, evaluations of people in the ward were socially constructed in relation to a complex web of powerful social influences. Key threads in the web are power and status, the management of uncertainty and negotiation through which evaluative labels become flexible and changeable, depending upon the social context. This argument is effectively a refutation of the dominant view in previous nursing literature, which is that personal biographical variables such as diagnosis or social class are in some way predictors of particular forms of evaluation of social value or worth. What now follows is concerned with describing and exploring what I will term social judgement from a theoretical point of view.

Towards a definition

By the term social judgement I mean the apparent judgement of the social worth of one person by another. The phenomenon is widespread, and all

92

humanity is involved in the process more or less continually. Judging persons to be good or bad may be nothing more than a human entitlement to appreciate, indeed to prefer, those aspects of a person's behaviour or makeup which we have learned to value. Another way of thinking about this is in terms of the respect we accord to persons. Leaving aside the question of who (or what) qualifies as a person, and therefore for the respect that ought to be accorded to them, the varying value which humans accord to each other is central to considerations of moral action. John Harris argues that:

> We show how we value others as much by the way we treat them as by the price we are prepared to pay, or the efforts we are prepared to make, to save their lives. (Harris, 1985:2)

Harris's discussion of the value of life is in the context of generally weighty moral dilemmas often provoked by advances in medicine. However the notion of variability in attribution of value to individuals has import across the range of health care delivery.

I think that at a theoretical level the term social judgement is preferable because it has within it the possibility of variation and change which other concepts, widely used, do not have to the same extent. *Good* and *bad* are useful descriptors, but betray any notion of subtle variation in an individual's label, and in variability between individuals. The terms also suggest an objective state in which the label very closely approximates the 'true' character of the person to whom the label is attached. Similar problems exist with the widely used terms *popular* and *unpopular* patients. Useful in one sense, as summaries of a supposed group consensus on the social value of a person, these terms have also the limitation that they really describe an outcome, for example that someone is liked or disliked. The focus of my interest is in the process and so the concept of central concern in the argument is that of social judgement. Restated in other words, I take this to be the judgement and labelling of the social worth of a person.

It is important to note here that a number of sociologists such as Roth (1972) and (Barbara) Johnson (1987) have used the term "moral evaluation" to describe this particular type of labelling. To those with a philosophical training this has a meaning more akin to the systematic philosophical analysis or evaluation of ideas or actions. I therefore suggest that in this analysis the term *social judgement* is preferable, if not completely satisfactory. From time to time, and in the relevant context I may utilise the terms interchangeably to mean what I describe as social judgement.

The term 'moral' in moral evaluation may suggest quite a degree of seriousness to a social judgement of someone. Assumedly people will inevitably express preferences about and between all sorts of phenomena in the world. Some of these preferences might be termed aesthetic, that is they suggest that one thing is judged superior to another, but there are no apparent moral consequences of such an evaluation. My discussion will however assume that wherever a judgement is made about the relative merit of a person then a "moral consequence" is at least possible, if not universally then at least frequently. Such a position is consistent with Harris (1985) and Wright (1971).

Social judgements, as may be already clear, may be negative or positive, that is people may be accorded a higher or a lower social value. A nice patient, a good lad, a lovely man, are some of the many examples of positive evaluations. A pain, attention-seeking, demanding, manipulative: these were some examples of labels used by participants in the study which suggested a negative evaluation had taken place.

Labels were not permanent in the sense implied by Stockwell (1972) when she claimed to have "devised a means of identifying popular and unpopular patients..."(p10). I suggest that this claim is false for,among others, the reason that labels may change. That is they may be re-negotiated.

Plurality

Labels were also pluralistic. By this I mean that patients were capable of being evaluated on more than one level even by the same individual. Physically they could be unpopular because of the difficulties involved in performing their care, but interpersonally they were liked, perhaps because they were stoical or humourous. Labels were uncertain in another sense, that there was no true consensus over the evaluations. Frequently nurses would suggest that privately they really liked someone who had been defined elsewhere as unpopular.

Thus, in a sense not far from that in which Goffman (1961) uses it, people in the ward had a *moral career*. They would begin with a label which was the nurses' official view. The career would evolve as nurses responded to the person and gained more information about them, which meant that the particular evaluation would change over time or be context-dependent. From this perspective the concept of *trajectory* has also been used to describe the evolution of a person's social situation through time (Strauss et al, 1982,b). These concepts have utility in explaining the fragile and far from permanent nature of evaluations, but may suffer theoretically from their implication that there is at any one time only one perception or construction of such a career or trajectory. Of course this notion is also suspect since, as I have shown, some judgements were covert. That is, they represented dissent from the 'official' label which was more often evident in formal communications such as ward reports. Perhaps it might be reasonable to argue that persons follow multiple 'moral careers' in respect of the perceptions of those who relate to them. This does not mean that all such constructions have equal weight in producing consequences for the person so labelled. Some evaluators have more power to realise the implications of their construction, a notion which I will explore in some depth subsequently.

Universality

A key property of social judgement is its universality. In the context I describe all my respondents were aware of it and of their own propensity for doing it. Equally, I became increasingly aware of my own social evaluations of my co-participants in the setting: patients, nurses and others. This sense, in which I recognise that I not only evaluate the worth of others with whom I interact, but that I may also influence the judgements of others in the research environment, is naturally of concern. My judgements of others in the field are very evident both in my fieldnotes and in the text as I produce it. In particular I am aware that I judge the work of others, as it appears in written form, and that sometimes that judgement goes beyond their work to them as persons. I either like or dislike them through my respect for or opinion of their work. I sometimes feel that this is wrong in research if not other spheres of human endeavour, but in pursuit of reflexivity I wish, at this point in my understanding of the notion, to make such issues explicit.

Assessing and being assessed

Assessing has become known among nurses as an essential skill, one which is described widely as the first stage of the *nursing process* (Kratz, 1979). Usually this particular activity has a specific focus, such as *activities of living* (Henderson, 1966) where nurses attempt to elicit a data-base upon which to plan their future nursing activities. Often the *assessment* is a clearly identifiable activity, taking place after admission to the ward, done by an experienced nurse, and recorded in some detail in the nursing records on a nursing history sheet. The activity is analogous to, and no doubt copied from, the history-taking which the medical staff undertake at about the same time, and which officially at least, forms the basis of medical treatment.

Assessing as I describe it incorporates not only these activities but also a wider sense of gleaning information about people in a less systematic way, as happens in ordinary interactions. A recent study by Jan Reed and Senga Bond (1991) in which 'nursing assessments' were observed elicited categories which reflected the themes they illustrated. One of these categories was 'global' such as "they're all hopeless on here" (p58). The second was workload related assessment, which had as its focus the number of staff needed to complete nursing activities for an individual. The third included references to personal characteristics such as 'awkwardness' or 'laziness' of patients. This approach also defines assessment as much wider than the interview and completion of the nursing history sheet which is described in textbooks on the nursing process (e.g. McFarlane and Castledine, 1982).

I have consistently argued that the traits or stereotypes theory of social judgement is inadequate. I do not reject the notion that pre-existing values and beliefs, or stereotypes, have some part to play in the social construction of social worth of persons in the ward. Indeed the contribution that social stereotypes make to the judgement of social worth is probably at its most powerful at the *assessing* stage, before patients and staff have had an opportunity to renegotiate the position.

In ordinary social life people commonly form first impressions of others they encounter. Roth's (1972) paper draws upon this notion, arguing that staff in casualty departments apply concepts of social worth common in larger society. By this he seems to mean that stereotypes are applied to the formulation of opinions about patients. He argues that this is especially likely in the casualty setting because patients are present only for a short time and a minimum of information is available upon which to base judgement. Roth notes also that earlier studies in longer term settings have shown that, for example, the young are more 'valuable' than the old (Glaser and Strauss, 1964).

Discussing the *interview as a social act*, and within a symbolic interactionist framework, Kuhn (1962) is keen to point out the social and cultural differences between social workers and their clients which manifest themselves in the social processes of the interview. The points he makes remain theoretically relevant. What he terms the interview for social workers, is analogous to the assessment for nurses. Applying his thinking to the nursing context he suggests that participants immediately have in their minds various questions which, during the assessment, they expect to answer. "Who is the nurse?; whom does she or he think they are?; with whom do they compare themselves?; who does the client think she (or he) is?". Kuhn goes on to note that Parsons' (1951) term 'affective neutrality' or professional detachment cannot really exist in such a relationship, since values and beliefs are inevitably brought to the encounter.

Kuhn sees the assessment as a performance in Goffman's (1963) sense in which participants present themselves as best they can. More than this though, they draw inferences from the encounter to construct not only their view of the other but to confirm or deny their view of themselves. In the case of the professional, they may confirm their authority over the client by controlling the interview or assessment process, and as Jenny Littlewood argues, by invading normally taboo areas of discourse such as bowel function. The patient, at the same time, may be confirmed in the role of passive recipient of nursing plans (Littlewood, 1991).

The process of assessing, which can be seen as a dialogue controlled largely by staff, is not merely a process of collection of biographical and medical facts to which stereotypes can then be applied, although this has its place in the construction of socially evaluative labels. Seen through a sociology of work perspective, the process of assessing takes on another dimension: that of the job interview. Because of the important but understated need for patients to contribute to the social functioning of the ward through work, broadly defined, they need to be assessed as to their abilities in this respect. It is no surprise to discover that the main agenda of the formal assessment process as part of the nursing care planning is focussed upon activities of living and the patient's dependence or otherwise in these activities. Such a model (Roper, Logan and Tierney, 1980) was the explicit mode of data collection on the ward. Other models make the goal of determining client's abilities to do the work of caring for themselves and others even more explicit (see the Self Care Model of Orem, 1980).

Strauss and Corbin (1985) address the question of patients being assessed for work in 'regimen management' in terms of their chronic illnesses, and other work by Strauss and co-workers (1982a) draws attention not only to the physical labour patients may be expected to contribute, but to the 'sentimental work' or what Hochschild (1983) and others (James, 1989 and Smith, 1992) have termed 'emotional labour'. These latter focus very much on emotional labour as a largely unrecognised aspect of the employment division of labour. Strauss et al (1982a), however, bring into view the considerable effort required of patients in the management of their and others' emotions. They suggest that patients are assessed and constantly re-evaluated as to their contribution to the division of labour in this respect. If they are perceived to be unable or unwilling to assist in, for example, the maintenance of secrecy (closed awareness) over a serious diagnosis, their ability to negotiate a valued social position is at risk.

Fineman (1991) develops the notions of 'willingness' and 'ability' to assist in (or comply with) professionals' views of appropriate care and treatment. In a paper discussing clients' 'noncompliance' with regimes in alcohol treatment centres, he argues that the staff do their best to assess clients for their intent in relation to treatment aims. This view, of assessing clients as willing or unwilling and able or unable, clearly has connotations of performance of work as its root. In this case the work is, for example, the preparedness to be honest, self aware, polite, open-minded and supportive of staff efforts (Fineman, 1991). All these activities for which the client is being assessed fall easily into a notion of emotional labour done by clients so that the analogy of the job interview is not so remote (Strauss et al, 1982a).

The patients' place in assessing

Assessing, as a first part of a process of social judgement is not something done by staff to patients. As I have argued, there is an imbalance of power in favour of the staff, and this means that control of the assessment of persons as socially worthy or otherwise is primarily in the hands of staff. However, an important secondary aspect is patients' awareness of the image they are presenting. I will argue later that negotiating and conflict or struggling also are main components in a theory of the process of social judgement. In order to negotiate or fight for their 'moral status', people generally have some insight into their current position. Indeed rendering this explicit can contribute to the staff assessment. One patient in the study, Nick Masters was able to invade the ward report to get analgesia on one occasion. On seeing new faces among the staff (such as mine) he helped to manage my first impression of him by suggesting "I'm not always like this you know!". By this I believe he meant to say that he did not normally break ward norms and interrupt staff. Charles Eastwood who had severe obstructive airways disease had considerable insight into how staff might perceive him as "a moaning old bugger like me". Patients may have some awareness of the outcome the assessment process may have for them, and as a consequence they make choices about the image they attempt to present. In the context of being very ill, or exhausted, as some patients are, the choices are confined by the practicality of getting through the day in comfort rather than presenting a 'positive image'.

Goffman's work *The Presentation of Self in Everyday Life* (1959) has a good deal to offer in the explanation and understanding of impression management. In his concluding remarks, he argues that '...as performers we are merchants of morality' (p243). Goffman explains this as meaning that underlying all social interaction there is a fundamental dialectic. This is that whenever individuals enter the presence of others, they need to 'assess' them, that is, they need to discover as well as they can the 'facts' of the situation. Indeed, both actors in such an interaction are party to both assessing and being assessed. The practicality of assessing is that all possible data are never available, so that we rely upon cues, hints, gestures and status symbols as predictive devices. This view seems at first to ally with the traits hypothesis of social judgement, but such a view is simplistic and fails to recognise Goffman's overarching principle that impressions are constantly amended and changed in the light of ever-changing definitions of the situation. This is so from both the point of view of the performer (in this case the patient) and the assessor of the performance. Indeed the notion of *performance* implies an active process of projection of an image rather than a passive possession of a trait or stereotype which may be observed by the staff and assumed to carry a particular social evaluation.

Assessing, then, forms the early phase of a constant social process of social judgement. In real time, any distinction between 'phases' of this process are artificial and for analytic purposes only. I will now discuss the climate in which social judgement takes place, before proceeding to 'negotiating' in my analysis of social judgement in the ward setting.

Summary

In this chapter I have endeavoured to identify and to illustrate the concept of social judgement. A wide literature has examined concepts analogous to this, calling them moral evaluation, social evaluation and labelling. My intention here has been to show how the concept seemed important both to my respondents in Howarth ward and to me as a participant observer. I believe that I show that labels are neither so predictable nor so invariant as the previous literature suggests. Particular features are that patients may be labelled differently by different nurses and that labels can be renegotiated, a point I will examine in greater depth later. I have tried to show how judging people is a key element of the process of assessing through which nurses begin their plan of care and through which they begin to control the moral destiny, or career, of their patients. In the next chapter I will address aspects of the context in which social judgement takes place. That is to say the social or organisational 'climate' for social judgement.

7 The climate of social judgement

I will now illustrate some aspects of the climate in which the application of good and bad labels occurs. It is from this point in my discussion that it should become increasingly clear that previous influential explanations of evaluative labelling have naively assumed that the origin of the label lies in patients rather than nurses. That is to say, the patient's medical condition, behaviour or attitude has been thought to be the chief determinant of an evaluative label, whether 'good' or 'bad'. In Kelly and May's (1982) discussion of the literature to that date, they summarise the conditions which had been said to give rise to labels, noting that they are all characteristics of clients or patients. They go on to suggest that work needs to be done to seek a more interactive explanation. Simply by assuming an interpretative (or symbolic interactionist) perspective in analysing the previous literature they became aware of its theoretical and methodological insufficiency.

It was clear to me very soon in my fieldwork, however, that these earlier studies had made important suggestions. Unpopularity did exist, and it was a cause for concern among staff and to some extent the people on the ward for treatment. Indeed patient characteristics, in the sense of the relatively immutable and non-negotiable, did seem to carry some weight. On a number of occasions I read a fieldnote or memo of my own, only to find an almost verbatim equivalent in Fielding's (1986) book, which I had not read before beginning my analysis. Here is an example from a ward report:

Raymond Lewis, aged 87 years. Has carcinoma bladder and dyspnoea, and has a catheter in situ "draining nasty-looking urine". Elaine (staff nurse) says he's "dead sweet" and "deaf as a door post".

Fielding (1986) gives the following examples:

Student: She's a very sweet old lady...   (p42)

and in relation to a elderly man:

Student: He's very deaf, he's a nice old man too. He's quite popular.
PF: Why?
Student: He's pleasant, always nice. Quite a character really. He's a real sweetie you know, a typical grand-dad. Dodders around you know. (p47)

My discussion will continue with an overview of what seem to be some of the situational determinants of social judgement. I will suggest that a key element is the power of the nurses and others to evaluate the social worth of their patients, that is, to apply an evaluative label. This considered there remain key categories in which this power is enhanced or reduced by local factors. It is convenient to discuss this in terms of situations relating to patients and nurses. There seem to be three overlapping categories in which the control exerted by patients over their situation may be discussed:

1. little or no control
2. some control
3. substantial control

These categories are of analytic convenience only and it is not my intention to produce and exhaustive review of possibilities. The ensuing discussion is meant to illuminate an aspect of the context of labelling rather than suggest its causes.

1. a) Minimal control: 'no diagnosis'

One patient I encountered was physically quite well. He was middle aged and seemed to keep himself to himself, being visited by his wife usually twice a day. He had been admitted under the care of a consultant from another unit, and complained of headaches and confusion. He would occasionally say unusual things, largely incomprehensible to the nursing and medical staff. He had a large number of tests such as a brain scan and liver function tests. Every test was negative or inconclusive, leaving the medical staff very uncertain about his diagnosis. As days went by, and then a week or so, a psychiatrist was consulted. This opinion too was inconclusive, that is to say that no proper medical or psychiatric condition could be determined. In the ward handover report I noted that the information we were given to manage his care was fairly minimal. On one occasion it was:

An odd man, not medical, not psychiatric. No trouble except when he's doing odd things. On haloperidol.

There seemed to be disquiet that this man may have an as yet undetermined mental problem, and certainly he seemed to have very little interaction with nursing staff. On another day he was described as "seeing things", in a way that implied that his symptoms were invented. There seemed to be consensus that whatever was wrong with Mr. Farnell, it could not be dealt with "on this unit". He was, as has been noted also with the elderly by Baker (1978), the right patient in the wrong place.

1. b) Minimal control: 'doing horsework'

If Mr. Farnell was a 'bad patient' because he had no suitable diagnosis, some patients pre-defined themselves as problematic when they carried specific diagnoses. I use the example of 'stroke' (cerebro-vascular accident, CVA) since this medical diagnosis was common and its features illustrate a situation which may prevail for other diagnoses. One of the experienced staff nurses, Rachel, was quite specific about it:

Rachel: People who've had strokes tend to be unpopular, because a lot of people who've had strokes, generalising, are very big and difficult to turn and they're usually, often, incontinent.

This view was shared by others. and was to some extent a consequence of the sheer physical toil involved in caring for some of these patients. One day I was responsible for the care of Sam Read, a very hefty thirteen stone man who had not long recovered consciousness from a particularly debilitating stroke. This required getting him out of bed, undressing him and passing him into the bath with the labour saving aid of a lifting device (Ambulift). This is described in a brief extract from my fieldnotes of the day:

...(Sam having just finished on the commode) two of us (then) undress him and put him on the Ambulift. We're sweating, me the most. Me because of the pressure I feel not being 100% confident and yet leading the care of this heavy and vulnerable person. After some fumbling we get the lift into the bath and give him a shave and bath.
The pan on the commode had a 'very good result' in it, so I feel much more justified in the persuasion (or was it coercion?) that I used with Sam to get him to have a disposable enema. I tell him, and he too seems happier but is still worried about doing more in the bath. I

shave him, cut his nose slightly! And then he does leak (faeces) into the bath and is embarrassed again.

We lift him out and dry him, mostly with an X-Ray gown. It's Monday morning and the laundry's late. We half dress him and take him back to the bedside covered in towels as the Ambulift allows his scrotum, penis and buttocks to protrude through the toilet-type seat.

With help from Olivia we manoeuvre him back into a big chair, and all this time I'm sweating profusely. I know it's both the graft, 'horsework' as Olivia describes it, and the responsibility of not looking completely useless....

Even in more practised hands than my own, this work is very demanding physically and emotionally. Sometimes, particularly at busy times, student nurses felt that even negotiating for someone to help with these activities could be awkward, as Susan suggested: "You've got to get someone out of the office to give you a hand." As a result of this, and the dilemma of having to disturb more senior or busy staff to get the work done, such work is stressful and likely to render patients who need it less popular, at least in this respect.

It now seems important also to note the presence of another situation of dual evaluation. By this I mean the possibility of carrying both negative and positive labels. Sam Read was a good example indeed. As a person, despite his need for fairly constant attention and his assertiveness in identifying his needs, he was undoubtedly popular. As a task, an item of physical and emotional labour, however reductive this view might be, he was much less than popular.

Kratz (1974) carried out a detailed participant observation study of the care, in the community, of stroke patients. Direct analytic comparisons would be unhelpful since by definition, even allowing for a shift in policy over admissions, most of her sample was not in need of hospital care. Nevertheless her analytic categories did include that of 'waiting to go into hospital'. Others were 'seriously ill', 'really getting better' and 'not getting better'. Of these, those patients defined as 'not getting better' were least likely to be highly valued as clients and to receive knowledgeable care. At this point of my analysis these concepts seem to have limited power to explain popularity and unpopularity. This may be because with other notions, such as medical diagnosis, they are but elements in a complex chemistry of social judgement.

Patients' social class, or perhaps more accurately, level of educational attainment, seemed to be a relatively weak determinant of evaluative labelling so far as nurses were concerned. Doug Whitbread was a retired bus driver who did not seem to obey the nurses' rules of good conduct yet, as I have noted, remained popular with them through a more subtle interplay of social skills and stoical and charismatic behaviour. Charles

Eastwood was a professional/managerial level engineer. Yet he was, at least as far as one could tell from ward and office discussions, very unpopular.

Although a detailed survey of the social origins of nursing staff would not have been appropriate, it was clear that those on the unit were predominantly of classes 1 and 2 (intermediate and professional managerial) of the widely used Registrar General Classification (OPCS, 1990).

In her interview with me, Anita (3rd year student) suggested that as far as she could tell social class was not an important factor in determining patients' popularity among nursing staff. She was less certain of medical staff however. Indeed she felt that nursing staff had a role to play in ensuring parity of access, particularly in respect of information disclosed by medical staff:

Anita: ...it's one of the things I like about nursing, nurses are more aware if other people are being prejudiced in the way they treat patients.

In the 1960s and later a considerable literature drew attention to the less than equitable distribution of health and other social care, notably varying by social class. A good deal of debate was engendered, but a number of empirical findings were not in serious dispute. Of particular interest was Tudor Hart's (1975) 'inverse care law' in which it seemed clear that availability of General Practitioner services more nearly reflected doctors' wishes to practise in comfortable middle class areas than to meet the health needs of the population, or indeed their claim to professional altruism. Other studies showed that patients of higher social class and educational attainment were allowed a superior interaction in medical encounters, that is, more time and better information (Cartwright and O'Brien, 1976).

Whilst Anita's view of some medical staff's equitable treatment of patients mirrored this opinion, she held a very positive memory of the experiences she had gained working with doctors in the Care of the Elderly Unit. She clearly felt that they did their best to give their patients all the options for treatment, with a full explanation.

This, however, extends the discussion to a consequence of negative social judgement, in this case of less information being given to patients by doctors and others. Whilst this link between social judgement of worth and therapeutic consequences is worth noting at this point, my discussion continues with an overview of the second category of social situations relating mostly to patients, but through which evaluative labels arise.

2. Patients having some control: being unreasonable

I suggested earlier that 'being demanding' was an unpopular label in its own right. It also has the broader meaning to the nurses of referring to patients who exercise too much in the way of personal choice or preference. This illustrates how it is that the meaning which attaches to labels is socially constructed. That is to say, meaning arises out of agreement upon usage by the people involved, in this case nurses.

Catherine, a staff nurse, explained how it was that patients who were demanding, i.e. challenging to care for, became demanding in the sense of unpopular:

Catherine: I think it's attitude really. You can have somebody that's demanding, but they're not necessarily going to be unpopular, you might 'tut' a bit, or say 'Oh, it's such and such', but if somebody's demanding and well, ungrateful sounds a bit patronising really, as if we expect someone to be grateful. If they're demanding you do your best for them and they're still not very comfortable, then you feel that you are not doing a good job. It's being demanding AND being unreasonable.

The imperative for there to be some overlay, some complicating notion such as 'being unreasonable' for 'being demanding' to qualify as a negative label, was also touched upon by student nurse Anita:

Anita: We've got a patient on the ward at the moment whom nobody seems to like ... he's quite demanding, in some ways unreasonably, but I actually quite like him, he's of no fixed abode and has had alcohol problems in the past. ...I dislike some of the things I have to hear about him.

Anita refers to a strong theme emerging from my data, that of (privately) liking the unpopular patients, and which I address in more detail in its place as a strategy for coping with the moral dissonance created by this situation. She does, however, validate the notion that being demanding varied in the degree of censure implied according to the degree of reasonableness or even thankfulness that patients displayed. One first ward student, Janet, made a suggestion that initially confused me. On reflection, I think now that I can see the sense in which her remarks illustrate the complexity of the social judgement of patients:

MJ: How about patients being unpopular, do you think some patients are more unpopular than others?

105

Janet: Yes. Charles Eastwood used to turn his electric razor on and just pretend he was having a shave. He was a bit inconsiderate.

I initially did not understand this answer, but she developed her point thus:

Janet: I think basically the patients are all in the same boat, the majority just want to get on.

She seemed to be identifying a duty to want to get well, to comply, and to co-operate with nursing care. Charles Eastwood was suffering from very serious respiratory distress, and was clearly very ill. What seemed to irritate Janet was his pretence at independence, something over which he presumably had some degree of control. As I discuss in the literature review, the notion of obligations of the sick to co-operate and to want to get well arise out of the 'sick role' which Parsons described in 1951. This model alone however does not fully explain the process of social judgement even insofar as the patient's control over the situation is concerned.

   Complaints from patients as from recipients of any service are rarely very welcome. It is, however, within the patient or client's span of control to decide to make a complaint. The limited, but best available evidence suggests that on the whole patients endure much suffering without complaint (English and Morse, 1988). Indeed not complaining is the norm in current British health care. One staff nurse gave me some insight into the problem in the context of our conversation about unpopular patients. Neil suggested that sometimes complaints were a symptom of another problem. He described his experiences of working with a young male patient whose constant complaining about apparently trivial matters was this person's way of dealing with severe pain about which he felt he could not complain. The patient was becoming unpopular until someone discovered his 'real' problem of pain:

Neil: ...but he didn't want to say that he was in pain because he was a big lad and it was wimpish to be in pain. Once we got his pain sorted out he didn't complain about anything.

This example illustrates on the one hand the difficulty for some patients of communicating their problems appropriately to nursing staff. On the other it betrays the 'wrongness' of complaining because Neil shows that 'not complaining' was the norm. Complaining is one form of interaction, or dialogue with ward staff, the initiation and therefore the control of which lies with patients. It can, however, be reasonably seen to have a function, a clear purpose related to achieving a worthwhile and understandable goal for the complainer, such as the improvement of some service or care, for example.

Another potentially worthwhile but sometimes irritating patient activity was that of asking questions. Again with the proviso that as an individual she both admired and encouraged this behaviour, Rachel (staff nurse) suggested that people who asked certain sorts of questions were often unpopular with the staff:

Rachel: Or the ones that question the treatment, the ones that want to know what drugs they're on, why they're having this... which is wrong.

A good deal of work points to the anxieties provoked in health care staff when confronted by either the potential or the actuality of answering difficult questions.

Melia (1987) discovered considerable concern among student nurses over their difficulties with this which, with other uncertainties in their work, she termed "nursing in the dark". By this the students meant that they were expected to care for ill patients but without either enough information or enough authority to discuss with the patients those things that seemed important to them. In my fieldwork it was evident that one particular patient, Jimmy Mackindoe, who had had a stroke and was suffering from lung cancer, was such a patient. Jimmy was making a stoical and determined effort to recover from the physical disabilities his stroke had imposed upon him, but the nurses knew about his malignancy whilst he did not. The consultant was initially determined that Jimmy's relatives' wish that he not be told should be respected. The nurses however were responsible for giving Jimmy morphine sulphate tablets, which he needed for his severe chest pain. Many people know, probably Jimmy included, that morphine is not a routine medication, and so the nurses had special cause to fear the most difficult question of all, "Am I dying, nurse?". As it was, Jimmy was managing his side of the uncertainty by 'buzzing for it'. That is, he was irritating the nurses by ringing his buzzer at or around the time the drug was due. Often this would disrupt the very nurse who was just in the process of preparing the medication anyway.

The buzzing was legitimate, that is he had no easy alternative way to let the nurse know he was feeling pain again, but for the nurses this was a constant reminder of a very difficult situation, one in which should he 'twig on' as one staff nurse put it, they would be 'nursing in the dark', not knowing what they could say to him. This was perhaps one aspect of a *process* by which Jimmy was seen as difficult to care for, rather than the salient feature being diagnosis alone.

3. Substantial control: "he buzzes although he can walk"

The third category of context in which labels arose and which could be generally attributed to some aspect of the patient, was that in which patients could be said do have considerable control over their situation. Of particular interest was behaviour which disrupted nursing work deliberately and without due legitimation. Robert Munro seemed to do this. He had tuberculosis which he had succumbed to in his life as a homeless alcoholic. Robert had been extremely ill, but was slowly recovering. At one point early in my period on the ward, Robert spent most of his time in bed, requiring assistance to move even in the bed. His degree of co-operation varied by the hour, however. He was unpredictable. He would invariably require help to move up the bed, or to change position, but then would be found lying on his back. Nursing staff worry, perhaps appropriately, that bedsores will develop when patients maintain a static position and are unable to move around the bed spontaneously as does a healthy mobile person. Robert was seriously malnourished too, another risk factor. The nurses' fears were founded, because he soon developed a substantial sore on his sacral area. A solution of an air filled ripple mattress was tried, but nurses still felt he was unhelpful in remaining in the sideways position in which he was put every couple of hours. This much is not unusual. Ill patients naturally find the position in which they are most comfortable, not that which conforms most neatly to the theory of pressure sore healing. But as my field notes reveal, Robert capitalised upon nurses' anxieties over his risk of pressure sores.

The experienced staff nurse, Irene had had an argument with him one morning over his refusal to lie on his side. She had been exasperated by his refusal not only to do this, but to let her examine his sacral area, which was known to be broken and deteriorating. At the handover report she had to report to us that he had demanded to see the Nursing Officer. Others in the discussion were sympathetic to her: "however ill he is, he's not as ill as he seems" suggested Rachel who reminded us of Robert's other 'manipulative' characteristics. As I have noted earlier he would ask the less experienced nurses to allow him his sedative (anti-withdrawal) medication at increasingly early times. Once one had allowed this, it became harder for others to refuse. He had, in effect, reset the nurses' clock. Despite the obvious gravity of his illness, visible even to the untrained eye on his X-Rays, it was hard not to retain some cynicism about his behaviour. "He's been playing this game for ages, both here and at North City Hospital, he's very manipulative," said Rachel.

Robert became something of a focus of nurses' emotions, either positively or otherwise, and remained so throughout my fieldwork. As he got physically better, he was able to walk around the ward to the bathroom, bathe himself with virtually no assistance, and watch television in the day room. He still presented a challenge to our patience however. As another staff nurse, Janice, explained, with some sympathetic insight into his motives:

Janice: He's always asking for social workers. Continually, and it's always for the same reason. He's been told, his questions have been answered, but he just keeps going over them, because he wants somebody to talk to. Somebody different.

She felt that he was lonely. He had few visitors apart from those social and philanthropic agencies which had a more professional interest in him, such as some local nuns. Relatives were said to have disowned him, and he had few friends. Thus there were many features which allowed understanding of his situation and his behaviour. Despite this, as there were other patients and issues to concern them, nurses found much of his behaviour irritating. Notable as a final example was his tendency to call nurses to his sideroom using the buzzer, even when we knew that he was capable of walking around the ward at his own convenience. The implicit rule was that buzzers are for those who cannot reach a nurse without them. I believe that as an 'experienced' patient, Robert knew this rule although he constantly and deliberately broke this and other 'rules' as tactics in a wider strategy of 'struggle' which I examine in detail later.

The climate of social judgement : discussion

It would be possible to locate a discussion of judgmental labelling at various levels of context. First there are socio-cultural factors which have a bearing, say, in terms of post-industrial European societies. At a different level the discussion could refer primarily to the British socialised health service and its principal occupational groupings and their clients. This study, however, is a ethnography of a particular medical ward in a large city general hospital. This means that I discuss mainly those phenomena which I believe appertain in only this specific context. However, this does not preclude the use of theoretical insights from other studies, however circumscribed are the claims made by their respective authors for their relevance. This section of the discussion will focus on power as a specific concept which greatly influences the context in which social judgement takes place. I will first discuss power as it emerged in my study and in relation to the health care literature. A main part of my argument will be that judgmental labelling is a key component of the maintenance of occupational power.

Power

I intend to show that social judgement is inextricably linked with the concept of power. In this section I will focus upon strategies used to maintain and to exercise power. In the concluding chapter I will address more abstract conceptions of power and their relation to social judgement.

In simple terms power is both the source and the outcome of social judgement. An awareness of one's own power to achieve goals through others is a fundamental aspect of the management of social relations. Terence Johnson's (1972) argument that professionalism is a social process, often managed in different ways according to the perceived power relations between client and professional, is helpful as a starting point. He argues that the strategies adopted by both clients and their professionals (such as doctors and lawyers) are features of a process by which power is both obtained and used. For the client negotiation is in pursuit of the service they require, and for the provider it is in pursuit of prestige, status and associated satisfactions. Johnson suggests that there are tensions inherent in provider-consumer relations which are controlled by means of an institutional framework based on occupational authority. His discussion is particularly apposite in that his terminology, two decades later, is highly relevant. These conditions apply equally to all occupations providing a service to clients, such as nurses in organisational settings.

Power, or in Johnson's terms 'occupational authority', has to be derived and maintained, indeed negotiated. The phenomenon of social judgement is integral to this negotiation process, that is, it is an essential aspect of the social construction of perceived power relations between clients and their carers. I will develop this notion by examining power relations, first focusing upon the role and position of patients.

Patients and power

It was evident from the analysis of my data relating to patients that responsibility for action and ability to control one's own destiny were in some way related. I identified three broad and overlapping categories, or states of affairs, in which the ability of patients to exercise control over their situation varied. These were minimal control, a moderate degree of control, and a large amount of control. Thus the degree of responsibility which patients were perceived to have for their actions was variable. This insight is far from new given that Parsons' (1951) concept of the sick role had within it both rights and obligations. These briefly are that the individual is not normally held responsible for illness and is exempted from normal societal roles. The obligations are to want to get well and to co-operate with medical endeavours to treat the illness. Jeffrey (1979) clearly draws upon these in his discussion of the typification in Casualty Departments of some clients as 'rubbish' because they break these 'rules'. I have already referred to the way in which some British sociologists have endeavoured to extend or modify this analysis to include atypical situations such as children in hospital (Dingwall and Murray, 1983).

I will argue that, whatever their merits as a starting point in the consideration of social judgement, such brief classifications as may be summarised in a two by two table must be inadequate to describe or explain the social and power relations concerned. In particular, the Dingwall and Murray (1983) paper, which provides the main account of this approach, does not seriously consider the strategies that are used by patients to modify the staff response to their deviant or rule-breaking behaviour.

Rather than patients' awareness of the commission of a deviant act predicting absolutely that they will be held responsible and receive sanctions such as negative social evaluations, I suggest that such a state is only a contributor in the establishment of power relations between the patient and the carer. Indeed being so aware can lead to patients realising that they need to utilise their other resources to redress the balance.

Patients' work

Strauss, Fagerhaugh, Suczek and Wiener (1982a) suggest that using a 'sociology of work' perspective can illuminate much in the social relations between patients and their carers in hospital. They identify the place of 'work' done by patients in hospital in providing a basis for negotiation upon other dimensions of social relations. Indeed they note the degree to which the social evaluation of patients by staff may depend integrally upon the nature of the work that patients are prepared to do. Strauss et al are at pains to identify in their very comprehensive paper almost all activities which take place in hospitals and in which patients are involved as work. They suggest that some work is officially recognised in the hospital division of labour, such as diabetics injecting their own insulin. Other work is not so recognised and may include patients reporting mistakes or deterioration in their patient colleagues. Of particular interest is the interpersonal dimension in which Strauss et al identify patients' endurance of painful or uncomfortable procedures as work through which the patient can then negotiate in other domains. Another area of work that they note is subtle but which if not done properly gets patients 'into trouble with staff is the case of the very ill person who knows she or he is dying. Strauss et al suggest that the patient is expected to do (unrecognised) work to maintain reasonable control over reactions which might be excessively disturbing of the staff's work, or disruptive of other patients' poise. Such an example in my experience was that of Nick Masters who knew he had lung cancer which had spread seriously. Nick was able to negotiate his way into disturbing a ward report to get medication, usually an unacceptable behaviour, perhaps because he was careful in his control of the more emotive consequences of his diagnosis.

This insight is useful because it also identifies patient work as a source of power, or a legitimate negotiating resource. It was a source of patients' control over their social situation.

Complaining

Groups of people subordinated in their power relations with others, such as patients in relation to nursing staff, commonly complain. Benyon's (1987) insight into patient's grumbling about medical and nursing staff, which he gained as a patient in a surgical ward, shows how much of this activity is evident, but informal or unofficial. That is, it is not directed at the accused. It happens mostly in the day room and is a source of relief of frustration among patients who commonly share discomforts and difficulties. Some formal complaints are made, however, and can present a threat to nurses who may perceive their image of competence to be under threat. The problem for the patient is often the judgement of the moment when a complaint really is the best course, in a context in which complaining can be labelled as 'difficult behaviour'. According to English and Morse (1988) in their ethnography of 'difficult' elderly patients, nurses said that "complaining patients made them feel they could never do anything right" (p28). Clearly patients do complain both about day to day things like the tea is too hot, or too cold.

Sometimes the criticism is more personal, such as that by Charles Eastwood in my study, who had apparently lost confidence in at least one of the junior nurses, Paula. Charles asked me, and in a way that others could have heard, to arrange for his care to be done by someone else as he felt that Paula was slow and clumsy. At one level he was expressing a legitimate preference, if indeed Paula had caused him previous discomfort. At another he must have assumed that reporting her to a nurse apparently in the rank of staff nurse might be a sanction both for her and an example to others.

This situation made me, as a nurse and as a participant observer, as uneasy as almost anything else I experienced. I was unsure of my responsibility to convey his feelings to more senior nurses and to Paula herself. Even more I was uneasy about my role in her defence. I

112

mumbled something about seeing what I could do (which realistically I knew meant me adding him to my own list of patients for that morning) but I also said something about being pretty clumsy myself at that stage of my training.

The point is that he had power over me, and Paula, at that and subsequent moments. I am confident that Charles had long since given up trying to be popular: his condition of chronic airflow limitation was too chronic, too discomforting and frightening to allow him to keep up appearances of 'niceness'. So in complaining he had less to lose, and something to gain. At least he did not suffer Paula's care which in his eyes was inadequate to his needs at that time. Such a tactic, however, is one most easily located within a concept of conflict or struggle, and is discussed in greater detail later.

Social exchange

Another attempt to restore the balance of power between nurse and patient is the exchange of services and to a limited extent of gifts. Officially discouraged from accepting substantial gifts, nurses are often offered small tokens of appreciation by patients. Sweets, chocolates and tights seem to be popular. Janice Morse, (1989) drawing upon the importance of gift-giving in the anthropological literature, suggests that the giving of care by nurses creates a further imbalance in an already unequal relationship between nurse and patient. Patients commonly wish to reciprocate by giving gifts to attempt to equilibrate. Whilst this notion may seem at first sight relatively inconsequential, the theoretical point is that the 'gift relationship' is a concept of some importance in the understanding of service relationships such as exist between patients and nurses. Malcolm Johnson (1975), drawing upon Marcel Mauss, argues that the giving and receiving of gifts is symbolic rather than economic. It is a confirmation of reciprocity that exists between individuals and groups. Johnson's thesis is that the elderly are frequently disempowered in these terms by being systematically excluded from the possibility of reciprocity, for example by being rendered poor and socially isolated.

Such a notion is not untenable as one explanation of the weak power-base of patients in the hospital ward. Generally the range of gifts available is small. Indeed it may be that the offering of such relatively insubstantial items as sweets is a modest attempt to fill the gap left by the minimal opportunity for a truly balanced exchange of services or other gifts.

Where 'patient work' in the terms of Strauss et al (1982) can be seen as an aspect of this 'gift exchange' idea, it becomes clear how those who cannot offer even this will be seriously disempowered in their negotiation of their image or their presentation of themselves as socially worthwhile.

I have discussed some of the climate in which patients derive influence to negotiate their social position on the ward. The analysis is not exhaustive nor 'theoretically saturated' in Glaser and Strauss's (1967) terms because my entree to the ward was in the role of nurse not patient, and so I claim less insight into the culture (or inmate world) of patients than of nurses. Nevertheless I accept the argument of Kelly and May (1982) and others that the patient does in fact have (some) power. I would confirm however that sources of substantial power are rare and little utilised.

Nurses and power

I now turn to an examination of nurses' power as an aspect of the organisational climate for social judgement. A large theoretical literature addresses these issues (see for example Freidson, 1970; Turner, 1987; Melia, 1987; Olesen and Whittaker, 1967). Here I will give illustrations of the place of nursing power and some of the means through which it may be derived in this context.

Nurses in the ward setting have access to considerable power. They use this in the daily lives of the ward inmates and it allows nursing staff considerable control over the experience that a patient has in the ward. Much of the nurses' power exists without autonomy however. Indeed much is delegated from another occupational group, the medical staff. Bryan Turner (1987) argues that the medical profession has exhibited three principal modes of domination over other occupations seeking to achieve the prestige and autonomy of 'professionalism'. In the case of dentists, the law was utilised to clearly circumscribe those areas of medical and surgical practice which mainstream medicine did not wish to deal with. This process was control by limitation, since the medical profession remain the arbiters of how much medicine may be practised by dentists in pursuit of their clinical or other objectives. In the case of the clergy and increasingly that of alternative therapists there is control by exclusion. Legitimate access to medical care is very much controlled by the doctors' function as gatekeepers.

In the case of nurses, Turner suggests that domination has occurred by means of subordination. Indeed he argues that nursing is "par excellence an example of the subordination of women to patriarchy and exploitation" (1987:149). He argues that the low position of women in the social structure has contributed directly to the exploitation of women's labour in health care as a direct reflection of the exploitation of women's labour in the home. Freidson's (1970) analysis of the power of medicine in relation to nursing remains useful today. From an interactionist rather than a Marxist perspective he shows how the authority of the nurse is dependent upon that of the doctor:

114

Legally and otherwise the physician's right to diagnose, cut and prescribe is the center around which the work of many other occupations swings, and the physician's authority and responsibility in that constellation of work are primary. (p69)

Freidson (1970) goes on to predict that, however aggressive the leadership of nursing (and other occupations), by being ranged around medicine these occupations cannot fail to be subordinate in authority and responsibility to medicine, so long as their work remains medical in character. The implication of such a position is that, to the extent that nurses have a high degree of control over patients, it must (whether they realise it or not) be in pursuit of medically desired goals such as compliance with treatment.

Nurses' power is in part also set in the context of a complex bureaucratic organisation. Whilst there has been substantial change towards professional managers rather than nurses with direct control of nursing, the control itself remains very strong. The position and influence of nurses in very senior positions was generally weakened by new management arrangements during the 1980s (Strong and Robinson, 1990). At ward level nursing staff still identify their line manager as a nurse, who takes administrative responsibility for several wards. Day to day responsibility for ward management lies with the ward sister/charge nurse. Still functioning as the central point for communication in and out of the ward on all important matters, the ward sister/charge nurse role remains, in this context, much as Pembrey (1980) described it.

Beginning with the qualified nurses, all had a very acute sense of their role in maintaining the dominant authority structure. One such example in the study was Irene, a staff nurse who neatly synthesised the relationship between the bureaucratic authority of senior nurse managers and that of the doctors:

Irene: I think... I would not disobey an order. One, out of fear of repercussions from the doctors and two, from my seniors, yes... because nurses are such a... In that respect it's very difficult if you make an error. You take something upon yourself whereas you're not a prescriber, as a doctor is. It could have very serious repercussions. You're not covered in any respect and you could be disciplined severely. So we have to tread very carefully.

In this interview we were discussing Irene's role as a qualified nurse in deciding whether to resuscitate a patient, and more particularly her perception of her authority to take a course of action other than that determined by medical staff, on contextual grounds. Irene was a graduate,

115

and a very able and articulate informant, but as can be seen she felt the power of the combined medical and bureaucratic forces to be overwhelming. Peter Conrad (1979) elaborates this notion with the term 'captive professionals' in which category he places nurses for this reason. As employees in a powerful hierarchical environment they find it difficult to act as advocates for clients. Rather, they are employed as vicarious agents of the social controlling function of the medical profession.

Thus, whilst subject in great measure to the power and influence of a dominant occupational group, nurses through delegated authority have considerable power over their patients. This power, though great, is fragile, precisely because it depends for its legitimation upon the dominant group and their advocates, the professional managers (May and Kelly, 1982).

Student nurses' power

So far I have described something of the micropolitical context of nurses' power in the ward. Student nurses were in many respects comparable in their influence over patients with the qualified nurses. They have the same general power to encourage, cajole, and motivate patients to perform the 'work' of being a patient that the qualified nurses did. In some respects however the student nurse's power base is decidedly weak. This, whilst self evident in relation to medical staff to whom they are virtually invisible, is most notable in relation to the qualified staff. Here I draw upon the work of Kath Melia (1987) whose analysis is confirmed by my observations in many respects.

Students see themselves as very vulnerable in their work on the ward. Melia describes how it is that because students are 'just passing through', they never feel a full part of the team, and therefore have to spend a good deal of their energy negotiating their place as people. They strive to be accepted so that the sanction of a critical ward report (practical assessment) will not be applied. They are aware of the informal power of permanent members of staff such as nursing assistants and domestics who may be on friendly terms with the senior staff. In the Australian context, Buckenham and McGrath (1983) make similar observations upon the lowly place of the student nurse in the clinical pecking order. Drawing upon interviews they summarise their argument as follows:

These student nurses, particularly the inexperienced ones, seem to learn very rapidly about the hierarchy within the nursing division of the health team. They are in no doubt about their own status within that hierarchy - they are junior to, and therefore more powerless than, all the other nurses. (p86)

116

Returning to the British context Melia (1987) comments upon the subtlety with which student nurses are controlled by their seniors. The formal sanction of the poor ward report was in many instances only the last resort. Senior nurses are able to communicate their approval or otherwise of student behaviour "with a look" (p19). Melia's informants talked of the need to demonstrate that they were "doing well on the ward", and the surest way of doing this was to "pull their weight". The look they got if they did not, was, I would suggest a hint of the 'social judgement' which was being or might be constructed around them in these circumstances by the qualified staff.

Nurses' power over patients

The power of student nurses in relation to their seniors was therefore very limited, as these brief examples illustrate. I will later discuss some of the strategies that students use to deal with their weak position in this context. In relation to patients though, student nurses have considerable power, given that much of this arises from association with the qualified staff. Students are authorised by the morning work prescription, usually by a staff nurse or above, to carry out those activities which the team and its leader have prescribed. It is perhaps easiest to conceive of the power so authorised by imagining the difficulty with which the insertion of a gloved finger into the rectum of a relative stranger would normally be achieved in everyday life outside of the clinical context. Most student nurses could achieve such a task within a minute or so with the minimum of explanation provided the social context, and hence the definition of the situation is that of uniformed nurse and anxious patient eager to conform to hospital routines.

This power, though in the main legitimated by reference to the authority of the qualified nurse to plan nursing care, (and thereafter by reference to the overall responsibility of the medical staff), is still very great. Jenny Littlewood (1991) argues effectively that the example of control of bowel and rectal function is not so bizarre. She argues that precisely because of the taboos surrounding the subject the demanding by nurses of information about bowel movements and their keenness to intervene in their production (or prevention) is a source of power over patients through the social process of humiliation.

It is easy to see the opportunities for control through humiliation that might arise. Such manoeuvres complement a wider range of strategies for control available to nurses at all levels, but their use by students illustrates their universality in relation to patients.

Other sources of influence

In order to further elaborate the context of social judgement I intend to proceed with brief insights into some of the other sources of nurses' power over their ward inmates. A nurse is usually responsible for making an assessment of the patient which guides the official plan of nursing care during their hospitalisation. As Jan Reed and Senga Bond (1991) observed in the context of the care of the elderly, this assessment is likely to make references to patients' personal characteristics of the sort that are not amenable to nursing intervention. An example they give is: "she's hopeless, she's just being awkward" where mobility problems were attributed to patients' personal qualities rather than functional incapacity of a physical nature. These observations mirror my own, and develop the point in Julius Roth's (1972) paper, that the first person to meet and assess a client is powerfully placed to have their personal evaluation of the person's social worth accepted as the starting point for future discussion.

The notion, popular among symbolic interactionists but not uniquely so (Merton, 1967), that a label applied early to someone becomes a self-fulfilling prophecy, is clearly relevant here. I have attempted to show how assessment, with its inevitable reference to stereotypes in the attribution of labels to individuals, plays an important but not exclusive role in the negotiation of social judgements made about people, particularly patients.

Power and communication channels

Another source of substantial power that the nurses control is the main information channel in the ward. Medical staff spend relatively little time with patients, and then are often accompanied by a senior nurse as mediator. Nurses control the main communication media in the ward, these being the ward telephone, the postal system, the major locations in which patient related information is discussed, such as sister's office, and the nurses' station. The nurses are also responsible for determining in many cases the rate and amount of information flow from and about patients because they control the events at which this occurs. I argue that the most important of these in the context of social judgement is the ward (change of shift) report. Research by nurses in the 1970s illustrated the great importance of the ward report in the decision process (Lelean, 1973). More recently Chadwick and Russell (1989), whilst discussing their observations of ward meetings in which a consultant physician was present, do ascribe considerable importance to this type of forum in exercising paternalism over patients in relation to discharge home.

David Field's (1989) thesis in his book *Nursing the Dying* is broadly that through their control of the ward information media and in their strategies of secrecy and maintaining 'closed awareness', nurses intentionally deprived patients of vital information in relation to their diagnoses, and perhaps more importantly their prognoses.

Two examples may confirm the notion in relation to the context I describe. In the study I asked third year student Susan whether patients got enough information on which to base their decision about acceptance of treatment programmes:

Susan: No... Not necessarily because they're not given it, in most patients they don't want it, they don't want to know. But I don't think there's enough provision to work out whether they want to know.

Susan seems to accept that the staff control the information flow to patients but is optimistic that with an improved mechanism for discussing such matters the patient might get to know more. Staff Nurse Irene, however, was a little more pessimistic about this. She was very aware that the authority of the nurse was dependent upon the wishes of the medical staff, in this respect especially of diagnosis and prognosis disclosure:

Irene: I think that's definitely a trait from the doctors. I think the nursing staff would definitely tell them more. But again we're not quite sure what we're allowed to tell the patient.

Irene illustrates my point well. The nurses' authority for action derives principally from the association with and control by the medical staff. However, as the day to day managers of sensitive information, the nurses effectively disempower patients by failing to release it. That they do this in the interests of the medical staff, and sometimes relatives, does not weaken the argument that they remain all-powerful in relation to the patient, the person to whom the information primarily relates.

Here it is useful to comment upon the notion of uncertainty. It is clear from the illustrations provided by Susan and Irene that the strategy of secrecy is utilised by nurses to manage their own uncertain position in relation to their authority to disclose important information to the inmates. The concept is also useful in terms of the maintenance of power by the creation and perpetuation of uncertainty in the patients about their illness status. The nurses' tactics for sustaining their own power base help to maintain their authority over patients in a less fragile form for other aspects of nursing care over which they themselves are more certain, such as, for example, bathing and the management of faecal and urinary elimination patterns. Control over these has, in its turn, the possibility for disempowerment through humiliation as I suggest in common with Littlewood (1991).

In order to use these tactics the nursing staff must necessarily control the important information channels even though they may not be the originators of the information, such as diagnosis or prognosis. I will later argue that, despite its complexity, there is essentially a close relationship between this control and the judgement of social value of patients by nurses and others.

Summary

In this chapter I have tried to document aspects of the social climate in which judgemental evaluations of patients take place. The differential access to and utilisation of power is a vital factor in this context. I therefore spend some time discussing both the way in which patients and nurses vary in their access to power, and the way in which labelling may be a vital part of the web through which the status and power differentials are maintained. In the following three chapters I will endeavour to continue my account of social processes through which I suggest that judgemental labelling takes place. Each phase of this process is overlayed by the concept of power as should become even more evident. I begin with 'negotiating'.

8 Negotiating

The negotiation and renegotiation of social reputation is complex. It is clothed within the dialogue and the actions, in other words the dialectical relations between all participants on the ward. It is also enmeshed within a complex relationship between the need to establish and maintain 'moral status' and the need to satisfy basic needs, wants and preferences of life as a participant on the ward.

"I'm not always like this"

Patients were aware of the need to negotiate with staff. Always there was an awareness of the considerable power of the staff to define appropriate behaviour. One patient with whom I found it both easy and difficult to talk was Nick Masters. He was about 55 years old, very articulate and generally interested in what was going on around him. He was quite rightly unsatisfied until he knew much more than the usual about my research role and my consequent interest in his views. Nick, I now know, was dying of lung cancer. I believe I knew it within a few minutes of meeting him for the first time, because he had ventured into the ward office during the report at 1pm and asked for his pain killer. Interrupting report was discouraged, but somehow the sympathetic way that the staff nurse stopped talking and gave Nick his strong analgesia told me he was either important or dying. Nick, noticing new people in the office, of whom I was one, said "I'm not always like this you know." "He gets himself into such a state" said the staff nurse, as Nick left to return to his bed. "He's been sweating lots since his DXR (deep X-ray therapy) and has a red area," she continued. By red area, she meant the tell-tale damage to the skin over the target area in the lung and caused by the X-rays.

Nick seemed to know he was taking a risk in disturbing the report, but also judged that he had good reason to deserve sympathy. I felt at the time that he seemed very aware of his situation, and resolved to talk to him if I could. Later we did converse, at some length on a number of matters, and Nick's decision to have vigorous X-ray treatment was of particular concern. He was very aware of unpopularity as a phenomenon, and one to be avoided if at all possible. He gave me an example of a time when one of his children was in hospital and he had demanded information from staff in a way that made the child, let alone him, unpopular. Now he tied this notion to his decision to pursue active treatment:

Nick: They offer you the treatment and you've more or less got to have it - what else do you do?

Nick seemed to be aware of the fine line between being 'demanding' and making reasonable requests of the nursing staff. He was also aware that compliance with the suggested medical treatment might be a factor in popularity with ward staff. He was, in this context, negotiating for relatively small concessions, such as analgesia on demand, by complying with major recommendations such as the X-ray therapy. Such a conclusion may oversimplify the factors involved, but has some merit as an illustration of negotiation.

Negotiated order

Negotiated order is a central concept in interpretative sociological thought. A famous paper by Strauss et al (1963) summarises some aspects of this thinking with particular application to rules and policies said to exist in hospitals. Strauss et al suggest that very few decisions are bound by rules as befit popular notions of bureaucratic organisation. They argue that actions and decisions assumedly appropriate to certain roles (as in a modern job description or role specification) are rarely so clearly demarcated. Rather, decisions are taken and actions carried out as the result of bargaining or negotiation between those involved. Such a view has interesting implications, such as for example that nursing staff take on activities and make decisions appropriate to both those above and those below them in the official hierarchy. Indeed, they argue, the modern hospital with its complexity of tasks and activities could not function without this degree of flexibility.

I will now outline some analytically important aspects of the process of negotiating in relation to social judgement. Strauss et al (1963) suggest that:

... a significant aspect of hospital organisation is missing unless the clients' negotiation is included...It is especially worth emphasising that negotiation - whether characterised as 'agreement', 'understanding','contract', 'compact', 'pact' or some other term - has a temporal aspect, whether that aspect is stated or not by the contracting parties. (pp400 - 401)

Negotiating in this context is the process of arriving at a working definition of a given situation. One aim is the negotiation of the social value of individuals. The process also involves agreeing the social relations, activities and roles to be undertaken or played out. This may include the 'tasks' or work of both caring and being cared for, that is 'sentimental work' or 'emotional labour' as well as the more visible labour of care. Negotiating parties are or should be aware of the sources of their power, so that their bargaining may be effective. As I have already suggested, however, patients are generally less able to utilise power than their carers who have far greater access to professional knowledge, information and other resources. Nevertheless the bargaining which occurs is evident enough, and usually is the antecedent of less amicable relations which sometimes arise when parties to the process of caring do not arrive at common ground or share (however temporarily) mutual goals.

"Go and negotiate"

On one occasion I was pushed into 'negotiating' with Ronald Byrne, an elderly Irishman with rheumatoid arthritis. The conscientious but perhaps underconfident staff nurse, Catherine, caught me in the middle of the ward whilst she completed her round of drugs after lunch. My fieldnotes record my dilemma:

"Go and negotiate with Mr. Byrne and get him to accept that he can't have an ambulance to go home in", said Catherine. It had been decided that he was to be allowed home that day, but had said to Catherine that he wanted an ambulance. It seemed that ambulances required 24 hours' notice, and I sensed that Catherine felt that Mr. Byrne could get home without one. To me he looked mobile but uncomfortable on his feet, so I felt awkward reasoning with him that an ambulance was unrealistic if he really wanted to go home the same day. He argued that he was a pensioner and that a taxi would be expensive for the three miles to his home, but I stuck to my orders and he capitulated.

This situation made me feel very uncomfortable. I understood, even if I did not necessarily agree, with Catherine's reasons for her decision. I wondered, however, why it was that she wanted me, a relative part-timer to do the negotiation. Later both she and Fiona confirmed my view, "He'll take it better from a man," they suggested. This statement seemed to confirm that it *was* a negotiation, that is to say that Mr. Byrne did have a chance of getting his own way. To avoid this, Catherine mobilised my gender (and perhaps my age) to add to the already considerable source of imbalance in the power relations between Mr. Byrne and ourselves, the nurses. Of course I felt uneasy about my role in this, and this example illustrates a moral dilemma for both more junior nurses and participant observers in the management of care where the need to co-operate with colleagues conflicts with a personal view about a patient's entitlements. This and other incidents have sensitised me to what I perceive generally to be a neglected area of moral dilemmas of intervention in clinical and participative research and which I discuss more fully elsewhere (Johnson, 1997).

To exemplify the process of negotiating in all its detail presents difficulties. One of these is that the specific focus of my observations was the staff, given that I was in the role of staff member not a patient. To argue that my insights are those of the patients by direct experience is therefore beyond my data. My observations may however supplement the work of others in key respects. Another difficulty is that sometimes negotiations are explicitly about some practical aspect of ward life, such as gaining medication or being allowed to forego a bath. This bargaining is overlaid by the constant awareness by both parties that their social worth is also negotiable, and may be enhanced or deteriorate as a result of the encounter. Therefore at one level of analysis all relationships are potentially ones where the 'moral career' of those engaged may be changed.

On another occasion Charles Eastwood who was debilitated with Chronic Airways Obstruction was discussed in the ward handover report:

He wanted a 'manual' (an evacuation of the bowel done by hand), he's had it and he's much happier now. He's got himself out of bed and he's really making an effort.

Clearly Charles Eastwood had been able to negotiate to have this done by agreeing to get out of bed as his side of the bargain.

Experienced staff nurse, Rachel, first of all typified the patients most likely to become unpopular as those who were physically hard to care for, such as heavy stroke patients. Clearly such people are immediately disadvantaged in any 'social exchange' because they incur so much physical and emotional labour. She went on however, to say that otherwise unpopularity arose out of patients' failure to accept nurses' definitions of the care they needed:

Rachel: Yes. The ones that don't play the game, if you like, they're the unpopular ones. The ones that want a bath when they want one instead of when you want them to have one.

Rachel seemed to be suggesting that unpopularity was often the result of failed negotiations between staff and patients. She went on to explain how it is that she would sit down and explain why she thought the bath was necessary, but also argued that she had a role in protecting the patient from becoming 'smelly' and that in some circumstances she would insist.

The example is relevant because it illustrates the continued, if in my view slightly weakened, emphasis on absolute control by nurses of patients' hygiene. This control automatically implies the potential for dirtiness and seems to be an effective strategy for maintaining the 'moral high ground' in that and other negotiations. Paradoxically, as I have illustrated earlier, the 'dirtiest' patients could also be the best liked, but this was because they had other personal qualities, such as charisma or a sense of humour with which to bargain for their moral status. Indeed to hypothesise a model of moral status with more than one dimension would be entirely consistent with this situation. In terms of the norms and taboos regarding cleanliness patients such as Doug. Whitbread, who was constantly covered in cigarette ash, they might be seen as 'bad'. In other respects and on the interpersonal dimension they might be evaluated more positively.

Fineman (1991) develops the concept of negotiation in the context of the counselling of alcoholic clients as follows:

> Staff members understood their interactions with clients as negotiated contractual agreements. Contracts defined by the nature and extent of interactions between staff and clients and specified the responsibilities and obligations of both parties.... (p357)

Fineman goes on to explain that not all the staff he interviewed agreed that negotiation was so consensual. One of his respondents, a nurse, told him: "I feel that we negotiate with them but I'm not sure that they do." (p357) This point reinforces the notion that the staff are bound to have the upper hand in any negotiations and particularly in the application of a label as a result. For Fineman the important labels were to do with staff perceptions of the clients' potential for compliance with treatment regimens. These labels included able and unable, willing and unwilling. His conclusion is that these labels are value-laden and are socially constructed. The comparison with 'good' and 'bad' is therefore not obscure and illustrates the close relation between the negotiation of day to day practicalities and social judgement.

Although it seems that many more recent investigators (Stockwell, 1972; Lorber, 1975; Fielding, 1986) have lost sight of the importance of an interpretative stance in the understanding of such phenomena, as early as 1962 Julius Roth was providing insight into the relationship between bargaining and moral status and which my observations confirm:

> Most bargaining ... is a product not of overt demands and pressures but of the anticipation by the parties involved of the likely or possible consequences of certain behaviour on their part... (p579)

He goes on to argue that:

> At the same time... patients..may try to improve their bargaining position by making a point of appearing 'co-operative' - telling the doctor how anxious they are to follow (his) advice, carefully hiding violations of activity restrictions from the nurses, and so forth - on the assumption that a 'good' reputation will enable them to win earlier privileges. (p584)

Roth was discussing his experiences both as a patient and as a participant observer in a tuberculosis sanatorium in the 1950s. The overlap between the two agendas for the negotiations remains as certain now and is just as difficult to separate analytically. Most of all it remains important to explore its meaning.

In one of their papers examining 'sentimental work' in hospitals, Strauss et al (1982b) firmly address this relationship. The first of their seven categories of sentimental work is 'interactional work and moral rules'. By this they mean that staff are responsible for maintaining their behaviour within agreed or negotiated limits. They argue that if certain taken-for-granted norms and understandings are violated then they will be classified by the patients as unhelpful or worse:

> Anyone who shatters those implicit rules or understandings is going to get, pronounced or otherwise, reacted to as inconsiderate, discourteous, rude, unpleasant, even brutal. (p259)

They are making the point that the staff have to do 'interactional work', that is to employ social and interpersonal skills in order not to be perceived negatively. This may be so for the staff, but I would suggest that patients have to work harder to maintain their positive image because they have less to bargain with and more to lose from having a negative label. Strauss et al (1982a) recognise this, however, and emphasise the

126

degree to which patients have to offer 'sentimental work' or 'emotional labour' in order to bargain for their moral status or social position. An example they give of coaxing someone to tolerate an uncomfortable procedure is very relevant and summarises the point well:

...or the staff may attempt to negotiate; 'if you endure it then we will do it as fast as possible' or 'only one more time'. (p979)

They discuss this type of negotiation, relating that if the patient remains recalcitrant then a negative reputation will build up. Strauss et al argue that the staff judgements about the cooperativeness of patients very often have a 'strong moral coloration'. This is because they involve not only someone's capacity to endure but whether or not the individual has the character to endure the procedure. My own observations confirmed the idea that patients are very concerned on the whole to maintain a positive reputation, and that this in itself is something to bargain with. There is an analogy with participant observation itself in that the investigator endures unpleasant aspects of the work in order to bargain for data, or at least acceptance.

The view that most roles and activities are negotiable rather than static carries within it an implicit critique of functionalist accounts both of organisations (such as Weber, 1947) and of roles. Explanations vulnerable to this interactionist critique are, for example, that of the doctor and the sick role assumed by the patient with fairly inflexible rights and obligations (Parsons, 1951). More recent accounts of patient-nurse interaction may also be susceptible to such a criticism, such as the study of factors influencing nurses' verbal communication with cancer patients by Wilkinson (1991).

Wilkinson's study used a variety of methods such as self report questionnaire, interviews and tape-recorded nursing histories, and is classified by the investigator as an analytical relational survey. The analysis is largely based upon tapes of the initial nursing assessment and from what nurses wrote that they would say in response to certain 'vignettes' or hypothetical cases. Wilkinson concludes from these data that among nurses who work in cancer care there are some who generally adopt the style 'ignorer' and some who are generally 'informers' in relation to their communication style. Collecting data from only the assessment interview which represents a very small portion of interaction with patients during their hospital stay is of course one weakness in relation to the conclusions drawn. The other is the use of self report instruments to examine what happens in the complexity of the real situation. It is clear that given the method and its perspective these conclusions are not unreasonable. What may be unreasonable is the assumption that nurses are so predictable and behave in the same ways so permanently as to be typifiable as 'ignorers' and 'informers'. The problem with this and other studies of a similar nature is that they assume a fixedness of personal skills, of human qualities, and of role-specific behaviour which is not borne out when the complexity of the situation in its real life context is contemplated. The concept of negotiation is in itself an immediate, fundamental and vigorous challenge to the orthodoxy which suggests that quantitative correlational analysis will help determine who is and who is not an 'ignorer' or an 'informer', or equally who is and is not a good patient or an unpopular one.

Wilkinson (1991) fails to recognise the importance of flexibility of response in ordinary and in professional-client interaction, and the importance of power in the context of and as a mediator of social relations such as 'ignoring people' and 'informing people' which do of course occur as part of the negotiated order of the cancer ward. As Anselm Strauss, (whose other work is extensive in the field of communication in cancer care) argued in 1963:

...the hospital can be visualised as a place where numerous agreements are continually being terminated or forgotten, but also as continually being established, renewed, reviewed, revoked, revised. Hence at any moment those that are in effect are considerably different from those that were or will be. (Strauss et al 1963:402)

Conclusion

Negotiating then, emerges as of central concern in the analysis of social processes which cause social judgements of persons as good, bad, popular or unpopular to be arrived at. Despite its early impact upon the interpretative literature of Goffman (1959), Strauss et al (1963) and others, the importance of negotiation is ignored by even quite recent analyses of social processes such as Wilkinson's (1991). Negotiating is common to most forms of social interaction between persons involved in the delivery and the receipt of health care. Where the strategy founders, or sometimes where it does not even develop, the strategy of struggling, remains as a way of achieving goals. I will now turn to this aspect of the social processes of social judgement in Howarth ward.

9 Struggling

Struggling is simply explained as the collection of strategies and tactics involved in attempting to satisfy personal goals in a difficult climate, whilst presenting an appropriate self to others. Patients who were mostly seen in a negative light were often aware that this was the case. Robert Munro, the homeless alcoholic, was a source of intense irritation to staff, as I have described. In the matter of his detention against his will on occasions, he too had cause for anger. One day during the period of tension when he sometimes expressed a desire to leave and to have his clothes ready to allow this, I was able to talk to him. In my fieldnotes I made a memo in which I identify a bargain he seems to have struck, which both sides honour most of the time:

> Whilst I worry that his detention is unethical, I think about his (Robert's) playing the game. Food, water, medication and (some) kindness for the duty not to run off (and get drunk). I chat to Robert and ask him what he will do when he does leave "I'll get a flat, I'll manage," he says, but then admits that he "desperately wanted a drink yesterday and I was horrible to the staff. They understood, thank God." This remark seems to imply his acceptance of the paternalistic restraint (not letting him have his clothes).

Here Robert clearly knows that his behaviour is not popular with the staff. He seems to accept their 'right' to detain him in what they perceive to be his interests. Nevertheless it is impossible to see the relationship between Robert and the staff as anything but a struggle. To entrain Robert's compliance with the staff's plan of care and treatment, coercive measures are used. Robert in turn uses hard bargaining skills to gain concessions such as getting his medication (to ameliorate withdrawal symptoms) earlier and earlier each day, preying upon the less assertive or less experienced nurses to achieve this aim. The social process here was clearly one of conflict or struggle, with deep emotions felt on both sides.

129

Avoiding

One illustration of the complexity of patient perceptions of 'required' behaviour, is that of specimen collection. Some patients are regularly asked to leave used bedpans for nursing staff to collect a faecal specimen to send to the laboratory for analysis. By far the most common of these is the FOB (faecal occult blood, used to test for gastro-intestinal bleeding which may not be visible).

When regularly reminded to provide a specimen for FOB, patients would conveniently forget to do so. One such was a young man, Kevin Peebles. He had a severe arthritic condition of the spine (ankylosing spondylitis) and was having X-ray therapy to prevent further degeneration. He had gone many weeks and yet the requisite FOB's had not been collected, usually three consecutive specimens. Compliance with nurses' instructions would have meant that he would have provided the relevant material. Nurses were, however, aware that he was "embarrassed" having nurses examine his bodily waste. Whilst nurses frequently deal with products of elimination of this nature, and most become desensitised to the usually unpleasant nature of this 'dirty work', it would be naive to imagine that the task is a desirable one. Whether or not perceived attractiveness has any part to play in patients' self-presentations, it seems not unreasonable that patients avoid the nurse's chief memory of them as being the nature and consistency of their faecal waste. Littlewood's (1991) paper provides insight into the social processes involved, noting that:

> When and where one may excrete in the modern West is rigidly controlled through laws...and the increasingly private act of excretion. (Littlewood, 1991:173)

Littlewood documents the sense of shame and degradation that people feel when the act of excretion becomes public. She argues that nurses are to some extent protected from vicarious shame by their 'symbolic purity', which grows out of their devotion to hygiene rituals and ceremonial distancing behaviour such as use of technical terms rather than lay ones. Littlewood's thesis is largely that nurses have the role of managing the patients' bowel function in order to encourage medical compliance through humiliation. That some patients try to avoid this humiliation, however much disguised as in their clinical interests, illustrates the weak consensus over these goals of care. It is as if patients such as Kevin are struggling for popularity, that is a more positive presentation of self, at the expense of their reputation for compliance on clinical grounds. In other words they are aware of competing strategies for achieving a positive image with nursing staff.

Conflicting goals

Other patients also had goals which conflicted with those of the nursing staff. For Sam Read, the elderly stroke victim, a goal was to maintain his dignity by being allowed to control his own faecal elimination despite his very considerable physical disability.

For Charles Eastwood the over-riding goals were to keep breathing, avoid undue exhaustion due to oxygen lack, and to keep to his strict routine so that he could maintain order in his uncertain and frightening world, perched on the brink of respiratory failure.

These goals were sometimes in conflict with other important aims such as the presentation of a positive image to others, notably nursing staff. Indeed then, one level of struggling is internal. It is the rationalising of conflicting aims in the changing social context. Individualistic psychological theories have attempted to consider such internal conflict in terms of concepts like 'moral dissonance'. The concept is analogous with cognitive dissonance in which diversity between behaviour and attitude creates a pressure for change in either or both of these variables (Festinger, 1957). Moral dissonance describes the same phenomenon when the behaviour or attitude has a moral component. An example from my fieldwork (which I discuss in detail in the chapter on *Aspects of Caring and Coping*) would be where, against my beliefs at an intellectual or cognitive level, I coerced Sam Read to have an enema. I changed my belief about the morality of coercion in that context because, having been asked to see that he had his bowels open, I was suffering 'moral dissonance'. I mention the context because I will argue that such individualistic (or reductive) explanations have only limited value in explaining my feelings or behaviour or that of others. In another context, in other circumstances, there would have been a different outcome. As one of many levels of potential understanding of 'struggling', however, the idea of moral dissonance has a part to play.

At an interactional level, patients struggled to present a positive self image in the context of expectations which were a direct threat to such an aim. That is to say, patients used covert tactics to maintain a more dignified image than their status as patients allowed. I earlier gave the example of the young man Kevin Peebles who avoided providing faecal specimens because the thought of nursing staff collecting and examining these was deeply embarrassing to him. In using such avoidance tactics he risked the displeasure of nurses who might be held accountable during ward round by senior nurses or physicians for the failure to complete tests.

'Being manipulative'

Another kind of struggle was that which arose between Robert Munro and the staff over a number of conflicting goals. Robert, recovering from liver failure and tuberculosis, regularly made requests of those staff whom he considered to be naive. The more experienced staff knew how to deny his requests or at least how to negotiate, to establish a contract whereby Robert would, for example, take a bath in exchange for being pushed in a wheelchair to the hospital shop to buy cigarettes. He had to bargain further for the opportunity to smoke them. So much was negotiation. Regularly, however, negotiations broke down and open struggle took place.

It seemed to me that because Robert was in any case a 'skid row' alcoholic, he had less to lose in terms of his reputation as a morally worthwhile person. He therefore more easily resorted to openly conflictual positions in his attempts to secure his aims. On the occasion when he had refused to let nurses evaluate the progress of his pressure sores (which he knew to make them nervous), he was accused in the ward report of being manipulative and the staff nurse warned the visiting house physician to "be prepared for hassle!".

Although Parsons' (1951) view of the professional-client relationship was one of constancy and agreement about respective obligations, the notion that conflict is inherent in such relationships is not new. From an interactionist perspective Freidson (1962) argues that "struggle between doctor and patient has gone on throughout recorded history" (p208). Although paying most attention to doctors, Freidson offers reasons why it continues to be the case that conflict is inevitable. These reasons also have import for other client-professional relations. First he suggests that objective differences in perspective between client and professional and uncertainties inherent in the routine application of knowledge to human affairs make conflict inevitable. Freidson locates the source of conflict in the clients' attempts to control what the professionals do to them. Freidson notes ways in which the professional (in this case the doctor) may forestall conflict, but recognises that each is problematic. The professional may completely accommodate to the demands of the patient, but if so, claims to professionalism are eroded. Patients may be informed and or educated in health affairs but through this mechanism they are likely to become more self confident and effective in seeking to control the professionals' work. Finally the professional may attain such high social standing as to gain an extra-professional source of leverage for controlling the patient. This, according to Freidson still leaves the client co-operating only superficially. They are likely to utilise covert tactics to achieve their conflicting goals. In summary and extending his own argument to cover other professionals he argues that:

It is my thesis that the separate worlds of experience and reference of the lay(man) and the professional worker are always in potential conflict with each other. (p209)

Clearly Freidson is at pains to illustrate the patient's role in any interaction as one rather more active and less predetermined than Parsons (1951) would have us believe. Given some attempt by the client to control both the process and the outcome of the encounter with the professional, Fineman's (1991) analysis of professionals' constructions of non-compliance is helpful. In Fineman's study professionals included doctors, nurses, social workers and alcohol counsellors.

Unwilling and unable

I have earlier briefly noted Fineman's discussion of negotiation in establishing co-operation with treatment regimes. His main analysis is concerned to show how it is that professionals take the lead in allocating clients to categories which each have a different moral status. Clients are, he argues, mainly labelled as willing or unwilling, able or unable, to co-operate (or comply) with treatment. These categories are clearly value-laden in the sense of being an evaluation of responsibility for, or moral worthiness of, a particular strategy the client has adopted in relations with the treatment agency. I find Fineman's paper helpful as it so clearly relates the integration between evaluative labelling and 'clinical' assessment. Fineman illustrates the phenomenon with a table of noncompliant behaviours (overleaf). Of course earlier I have criticised such simplifications, but it seems to me that Fineman's table represents a different perspective. Whereas Stockwell (1972) and others were concerned to label predictive patient traits and behaviours, Fineman's emphasis is that the categories he isolates are subjectively those of the staff. In his words:

Staff members sought to know and explain why their clients misbehaved. As a consequence, they subjectively assessed the intent underlying their client's misbehaviours. In doing so, they constructed interpretive categories that distinguished between those clients who were perceived to be unwilling to comply and those who were perceived to be unable to comply.

Table 3: Fineman's categories of non-compliance
(after Fineman 1991 : 359)

Unwilling	Unable

1. Manipulative
A. Sabotage
B. Working the system
   i) Doctor shopping
   ii) Seeking undeserved services
   iii) Provoking fights among staff
2 Recalcitrant; rigid; stubborn
	1 Physically disabled
	2 Cognitively impaired
	3 Alcohol addicted

	(see Fineman, 1991:359)

Fineman elaborates these categories in more detail, showing for example that doctor shopping refers to clients who recruited multiple staff members to work to contradictory ends. Sabotage meant agreeing to a course of action and then failing to go ahead with it. As it happens, Robert Munro's conflictual stance could be explained to some extent by our view of his behaviour in categories very similar to these. It was commonly the case that nurses would negotiate with him and get an agreement, say, that he would get up for a few hours in the afternoon if allowed to sleep in the morning. The nurse making this agreement, myself included, would feel that they had allowed choice and an individualised approach to his care. Later however, he would be found to have capitalised on a change of staff to avoid getting up (sabotage).

Fineman seems to argue that all categories of non-compliance are socially constructed, a position with which I have some sympathy. It could easily be argued, however, that some of these categories would be so widely agreed upon that they are for practical purposes 'objective' categories or criteria of willingness or ability to comply or co-operate with treatment. Nevertheless, his notion of the staff's understandings of clients' willingness to comply with treatment is worth considering. This is particularly because the staff's categorisation of the client in these respects "provided the moral and rational bases for the compliance management strategies they used," (Fineman, 1991:372). Fineman also gives some insight into some of the strategies for conflict or struggle that clients may use to manage their relations with professionals.

Conflict and social exchange

In a complex theoretical paper which draws heavily upon exchange theory, Blegen and Lawler (1989) also confirm the view that much of the client-professional relationship can be explained in terms of power and conflict. Their paper analyses the tactics used by low-power individuals to influence higher-power ones, and develops a classification of tactics which they suggest links the choice of tactic to the power relationship. Blegen and Lawler affirm that tactics available to the client are of two main types. First there are those means which utilise the existing power relations between client and professional. Second there are those which attempt to change the power relations.

In acting upon existing power relations the client can remind the professional of their official obligations, such as when patients remind nurses that their drugs are due at a certain time. Patients can threaten to leave, which can be embarrassing for staff to have to explain to their seniors. This was a tactic utilised by Robert Munro and by which the staff felt threatened enough to deprive him of his outdoor clothing. Robert also used the third tactic, that of threatening a report to senior management. The other tactic applied within existing power relations would be the direct use of a sanction, a punishment or a reward. Blegen and Lawler see this as a broad category including such as praise, insult or even bribes. Though broad, this category also offered patients on Howarth ward minimal opportunity to redress power imbalance since formal 'gift-giving' is an activity usually done on leaving. Criticism could be powerful, but most in relation to those staff with an insufficiently established reputation. Such persons were likely to be student nurses and participant observers bargaining for access.

Blegen and Lawler (1989) continue their theory of tactical action with analysis of attempts by clients to change the power relations, that is, to gain more power themselves or weaken that of the professional. They suggest that it is possible to decrease the authority's power by decreasing one's own interest in goals towards which the authority is working. To enhance relevance I offer the example of, say, the patient with an incurable disease who decides to be less motivated toward active treatment than palliation. Such a position disempowers the doctor and, in the typical medically dominated context, the other occupations who define their actions mainly in terms of active treatment.

A second, and it seems to me related disempowering tactic is actively to seek alternative goals to those of the professionals. This, Blegen and Lawler argue, can be combined with forming coalitions with other clients to reduce dependence upon the professional. A final tactic they offer is for clients to increase the value of those goal outcomes sought by the professional and provided by the client. Despite its at first abstract language, this tactic implies that the client controls to the fullest extent the outcomes of interaction sought by the professional. In private practice this can be by payment. Indeed this tactic could then be seen merely in terms of a shift in the type of professional-client relations from one of mediative professionalism (money only changes hands at a great distance through a remote bureaucracy), to one of patronage, where the client pays directly and usually can make greater demands (Johnson, 1972). The outcome desired by the professional may however be interactive, or qualitative, and to the extent that the client can present a self image which enhances this qualitative goal outcome for the professional they will possess enhanced power in the relationship. An example would be the client whose illness or behaviour is clinically interesting to the doctors or nurses.

To summarise, the client who can get to be liked will have the greater power, or be the least disempowered. Here too then, there is a complex but unavoidable link between assessment, interpersonal realtions and social judgement in client-professional relations.

Struggle and labour

The general perspective of 'sociology of work' has, as I have suggested, a good deal to offer in the interpretation of social relations in the ward, and this is no less the case in terms of conflict or struggle. Making clear the relationship between a patient's reputation with staff and their willingness to do 'the work of the hospitalised patient', Strauss et al (1982a) remind us that this work is broadly defined and includes:

> ...cooperation,behaviour that involves endurance, fortitude, self control in the face of discomfort, pain or potentially humiliating medical intervention. (p979)

Given that some patients seem unwilling to accept this division of labour or to recognise their role in performing such work, the staff will initially negotiate with them. When, however, these negotiations fail:

> The staff may cajole, tease, scold, empathise but insist on obedience; thus attempting to persuade the patient. (p979)

Strauss et al point out in particular that staff are keen to judge the actions of patients in carrying out this work, because, they argue, there is an implicit moral code to be followed. Indeed patients may "morally evaluate" their own actions as "being proud or ashamed at their endurance or fortitude" (p979).

To examine the social production of labour with an emphasis on the concept of conflict is to take essentially a Marxist perspective. It would be wrong to argue that Strauss and his colleagues have such a perspective in their work in general and in this paper in particular. Struggle in terms of class struggle is barely evident in any of their work. Some recent British work (James, 1989) addressing hospital care from a 'sociology of work' point of view does more explicitly draw upon Marxist and feminist notions of oppression, class struggle and conflict based in the economic relations between competing groups. Such analyses of hospital health care and other forms of work have tended to concentrate upon the division of labour in terms of the staff. The recurrent thesis is that 'emotional labour' (or sentimental work) is difficult to account for (both in economic and responsibility terms) and is culturally associated with low status groups in general and women in particular (James, 1989; Smith,1992).

To extend the analysis directly to patients or clients in terms of conflict over the division of labour is interesting but presents substantial problems. Much further work could be done in this area. However some exploratory questions are raised by such thinking. First it might be asked to what extent patient work of both a physical and 'sentimental' or 'emotional' kind is essential to the maintenance of care delivery and standards of care? Second, what is the relationship between ideologies of independence or self care and wider cost reduction initiatives in health care? Third, and of explicit relevance to my own thesis, would be how far the reputation of the client is affected by their capacity for productive work Reframed the question is: what is the relationship between the contribution the patient makes to ward work, in economic terms, and the social evaluation they earn and its consequences for the standard of their care?

Whilst little in the way of empirical work has examined these questions in health care settings, a good deal of theory has related to the notions of struggle and conflict between competing groups. Parsons (1951) saw client-professional relations in terms of consensus of goals. Each party to the interaction is seen to want the same outcome, and thus the concept of coercion, or struggle has little place in his analysis. Rex (1961) attacks Parsons' conception of social relations as essentially flawed for precisely this reason. In a general theory of human relations Rex outlines as its first principle the idea that:

Instead of being organised around a consensus of values, social systems may be thought of as involving situations at central points. Such conflict situations may lie anywhere between extremes of peaceful bargaining ....and open violence. (p594)

Rex argues that this principle should form the basic assumption in the analysis of social relations at any level of social system from wider society to smaller social systems (such as a ward).

Giddens (1968) seems at first more forgiving of Parsons' naivete arguing that in his later works he had at least drawn the concept of power into his theories. Giddens goes on, however, to show that in Parsons' conception of power it is seen as always legitimate, that is to say it is taken from a mandate given by those who may be subordinated to the authority of the power holder. To some extent this Parsonian conception of the power used in nurse patient relations may be accurate. By this I mean that in terms of the outcome, many patients and nurses would share the same long term goals. Where they may differ is in the means to achieve these outcomes, and it is here where substantial conflict occurs but which a Parsonian account would not recognise. The category of the process of social judgement which I have called struggling is arguably one which locates conflict in the means of delivery (or of acceptance) of care, rather than the outcome. Of course there are also areas where there is a clear difference of desired outcome of care and or treatment between client and professional. Such an example would be the different views which some patients may have from their doctors (and nurses) when being treated for a painful and uncomfortable terminal condition (McIntosh, 1977).

Whilst Parsons would argue that seeking and accepting treatment necessarily provides a mandate for professional authority, and therefore compliance with treatment, such a view is not supported by my evidence offered here. The social processes involved in care and treatment are more effectively illuminated from a conflict perspective, whether this is in terms of a general theory of human relations as Rex (1961) would have it, or in terms of the control and social production of labour in the ward (James, 1989, Smith, 1992).

By way of summary of the category of struggling and in order to shed further light upon the notion of struggle in the context of social judgement, I intend to draw upon the study by English and Morse (1988). Having used various qualitative methods to study perceptions of nurses and patients to 'adjustment' of difficult elderly patients, they suggest the following tentative model:

Table 4: Key concepts in the patients' model of how difficult behaviour comes about (after English and Morse, 1988 : 31)

LACK OF CONTROL AND POWER -patients made to wait -submissive nurse-doctor-patient -relationships -nurses judge, condemn -treatments/pain control -patient assertiveness	**EXPECTATIONS NOT MET**
LACK OF INDEPENDENCE -lack of knowledge -patient dependent role -elderly role -ask for assistance -lack of hope	**FEELINGS/EMOTIONS** -embarrassed -dissatisfied -pessimistic -abandoned -lonely -bored -let down, disappointed -resentful -frustrated -irritated -worried, anxious -afraid, apprehensive -angry
LACK OF COMMUNICATION -information not shared -old charts not read -non-response of staff -information witheld(control) -lack of teaching -no-one listens	**LEADS TO 'DIFFICULT BEHAVIOUR'**
LACK OF CARE -lack of respect, patience -lack of nurse advocacy role -nurse unreasonable -lack of communication -argumentative -nonchalant attitude	**LACK OF CONTROL OF TREATMENT** -drug reactions/side effects -drug errors -treatment reactions/side effects -treatment errors -incorrect procedures -lack of response to treatment/drugs

English and Morse (1988) do not expand very much in terms of the detail of these categories. However, they are at pains to emphasise that they see patient-nurse relations as a struggle between two opposed groups with sometimes very different goals both of the means and of the ends of care:

> In summary, the lack of communication between nurses and patients appeared to contribute to lack of clarification of patient role-expectation, increased patient anxiety regarding standard care, a perceived lack of care, comfort and respect for the elderly patient as an individual and a failure of the nurse as a patient advocate. Overall there appeared to be a power struggle regarding who was in control and whether the patient would be allowed to maintain (his) independence while in a dependent role. (English and Morse,1988:31)

This model, as exploratory as it may be in terms of its grounding in the relatively specific social context investigated by English and Morse, is nevertheless one of few attempts to present the patient perspective in the area of social judgement, if not nursing in general. It also successfully recognises the central point that struggling has in the social relations of hospital care.

Conclusion

In the discussion of struggling, I have outlined some examples of the tactic as utilised by patients and their nurses. I have attempted to integrate the concept into a broader discussion of the notion of conflict, as seen from a number of differing but related perspectives. These are symbolic interactionism, (specifically the sociology of occupations and work), Parsonian functionalism, exchange theory and the neo-Weberian conflict perspectives of Giddens (1968) and Rex (1961).

Each of these has something to offer the analysis, and this is particularly true of the concept of struggle and its underlying issues of power an conflict in social relations. Again maintaining the artificial, but I hope analytically helpful distinctions between the categories of the process of social judgement, I will proceed now to a discussion of acquiescing, the last of my chief analytic categories of the process of social judgement.

10 Acquiescing

Acquiescing: the beginnings of compliance

The final aspect or category of the process of social judgement as I discovered it is acquiescing. The concept seems to have a good deal in common with compliance, that is, it has to do with tactics and strategies through which people on the ward, and patients in particular, went along with the wishes of the dominant authority. "Going along with it" was a common expression among nurses and patients. The important distinction is that it describes a process, rather than an end state. Compliance, which may be nearer to an outcome of the process of acquiescing, has been a major subject of investigation from a number of perspectives. The medical profession often defines the success of treatment by the degree of compliance with a prescribed course of treatment (Brand and Smith, 1974). Treatments that the patient does not continue with may be seen as unsuccessful, and others are developed. Compliance is also important to those who allocate health care resources, an illustration might be the choice of persons to participate in expensive treatment programmes such as major organ transplant or dialysis. This is because it is argued that it would be wrong to allocate scarce resources to those who will not utilise them properly (are not compliant).

Sociologists have also had a major interest in compliance. In very general terms those working primarily from a functionalist perspective attempt to describe non-compliance as a deviant act, not in accordance with normative conduct, and therefore rightly and properly worthy of social control (Parsons, 1951). Interactionists have been more interested in how behaviour comes to be defined as compliant or otherwise. From a Marxist perspective, compliance is seen as the end state of social control through which persons are returned to their subordinate and productive place in the capitalist division of labour (Navarro, 1976). This position is fruitfully allied to the interactionist 'sociology of work' perspective, in that compliant patients are seen to be those who do the productive work of co-operating with treatment agents or assisting in their own care or that of other patients.

I recapitulate these points in order to clarify, as far as possible, the notion of compliance and its relation to the concept 'acquiescence' as I discover it. Acquiescence is "to rest satisfied without making opposition; quiet ascent or submission" (Geddie, 1964). Acquiescing is therefore a process of submitting to the will of others, of giving up a struggle (where one has occurred). It has therefore a different focus from compliance. It is, in one sense, almost a psychological process through which a person may go in deciding to comply.

I remain concerned that use of this term will be vulnerable to a lack of clarity and coherence. It certainly overlaps with compliance in some large degree, since this latter word can also be part of an internal psychological process of becoming compliant. In thinking about the use of language, it is worth noting as Turner (1987) reminds us, that the patient is "one who exercises patience". Patients could be seen to acquiesce to nurses' wishes in a number of ways. On the whole, they would get up when asked to do so. They would take a bath when encouraged to do so. Indeed the bath remains a focal point in the illustration of the control nurses maintain over their patients. There is more flexibility about this than previously, when patients took a bath every day. Nevertheless, the bath is often, as I have described, a physically and emotionally demanding activity for nurses and so even experienced staff nurses like Catherine did not want to suffer the accusation from their seniors that "You got out of it too easily!"

This therefore meant pressurising patients subtly or otherwise to acquiesce to their wishes not only to have a bath, but be seen to do so. Damp combed hair, a good shave, and clean night clothes were part of this imagery, which I too felt the pressure to produce in "my" patients. The new flexibility of individualised care meant that at least there was now room for judgement. Perhaps a strip wash at the sink could be taken instead. But eventually the pressure built up.

Complete trust

At the compliant end of the continuum lies the patient exhibiting complete trust. This is not so much a category of patient or person, as a strategy which any person may adopt. That some are more likely to do so than others may be true, but the strategy of complete trust is, like other approaches to the patient role, context-dependent. It can however, as in the case of John McGee, a person with septic arthritis of his knees and other joints, be a very consistent strategy. I record here a substantial portion of my field record of my impressions of Mr. McGee in order to contextualise the point I make as much as possible:

John McGee has had lots of hospital admissions. His wife is a nurse. He tells me something of his early medical history and his treatments in various hospitals around the country. He talks about male nurses (knowing I am one). "I've never liked them", he checks and looks at me..."until recently", he adds. He tells me that in his considerable experience they have the "wrong attitude. They don't smile nicely...whereas the girls, they always have the right attitude."
He goes on to patients' notes and the recent newspaper article (saying) that patients are able to see their "notes". "I don't agree at all, you should have complete trust in the doctors and nurses. They don't force you to come into hospital, it's your choice". He says that "patients don't understand medicine, nursing and the notes, so more harm than good will come of it."

John McGee went on to outline how despicable it would be for people to sue the hospital since they had asked for the treatment in the first place. At first I was unsure of the reason he was articulating these views to me, but it seemed that he did so to anyone who would listen. He hated the patients who seemed to be asking for things, and in particular saw it as his role to point out 'inappropriate' behaviour from other patients. It was Mr. McGee who first told me about Albert Littlewood's "weeing in the sink". John McGee was in many ways, then, conforming to his perception of the ideal patient. He had had a long time in hospitals to formulate his strategy. Even the apparent risk he took in criticising male nurses was located in his past, and in what I think was his idealised notion of the hospital and its perfect patients and perfect (female) nurses.

It was impossible to be offended by his views. They were based upon his experiences. He was compliant in the extreme, based upon his view of the right and proper superiority of the medical and nursing staff. 'Going along' was his *modus operandi*. I do not think his tactics are unique.

Mr. McGee could be described as almost 'permanently acquiescent'. Some nurses put this down to the older patients generally being more likely to see the hospital authorities as always knowing best, but others suggested that it was too easy to coerce any of the patients and that the uniform was a very important symbol of this power.

Other patients would acquiesce in some respects and not others, and here the concept overlaps with negotiation and struggle. Acquiescing could be more temporary, such as in the case of Sam Read's final but reluctant acceptance of the enema we gave him. We knew afterwards that despite the relative success of the procedure by our clinical criteria, he might be just as vigorous in defence of his autonomy next time. On the other hand, as Littlewood (1991) argues, we successfully defeated Sam on that occasion. Such a demonstration of our power would, especially in respect of the taboo area of bowel control and the nakedness required to complete the task, increase his vulnerability to nursing and medical power in the future.

In an ethnography of nurse-patient conversation styles in an Australian nursing home, Gibb and O'Brien (1990) show the degree to which nurses instruct patients in the course of daily care activities such as bathing and toileting. For me at least, the word toileting says it all. It is something patients have done to them, and there is little or no choice. Patients must necessarily acquiesce to this and to other ideas such as where they might sit. They receive instructions to this effect:

> ...it was apparent that nurse's inquiries regarding the resident's preferences extended only between a limited range of options. This was signalled through the repeated use of closed questions which required merely yes or no answers. Lack of any negotiation through the use of open questioning such as "Where would you like to sit today?" was stridently obvious. (Gibb and O'Brien, 1990:1398)

A recent small study by Hewison (1995) in a British elderly care area gave stark, if brief, examples of the use of language to engage compliance with routine care objectives:

Nurse: You'll have to put this dress on. Stand up, stand up (puts dress on patient). Sit down, sit down (spoken harshly).

Hewison uses other examples in which terms of endearment are used to engage co-operation with care and which, in print, seem patronising and demeaning mimicking language used with children. Reflecting on my own practice, I see myself here, using terms like 'poppet' and 'sweetie' with women who seemed vulnerable and in discomfort. Perhaps in some situations such language may have an appropriate place. What is important is that we become aware of our use of language and think more deeply about its implications. As to the harsher language with patients in our care I wish I could disclaim any use of it, but I would be lying.

'Toeing the line'

To return to the British context, I have earlier criticised the broad-based conclusion drawn by Waterworth and Luker (1990) from their interviews with 12 patients on different wards in a Liverpool Hospital. I suggested that they should not conclude too seriously that "...some patients are more concerned about doing what is right , that is, pleasing the nurse, than participating in decisions concerning care." (p971)

This is because they only interviewed people who met the criterion 'willing to be interviewed'. Such respondents were therefore pre-selected as 'trying to please the nurse', in this case the investigator. However, one of the chief categories produced by the analysis Waterworth and Luker (1990) provide is 'toeing the line'. They argue that their respondents' chief preoccupation was with 'staying out of trouble'. To do this the patients found it essential to discover the rules and exhibit the right behaviour. The patients interviewed were willing to relinquish their freedom and responsibilities in order to 'toe the line'. A second category is 'accepting the situation'. This, Waterworth and Luker argue, showed how patients are willing to comply with the routines and why some patients believed "they had no rights in hospital" (p973). Patients' passive acceptance of nursing plans is illustrated by a respondent's opinion about the difficulties they would discuss with nursing staff:

> You wouldn't grumble at the nurses, that's not fair, because in any case you are at the mercy of whoever. I mean it's like sitting in the dentist's chair, you know you couldn't say much if you wanted to. (p973)

This is an important point, because it shows that even allowing for the possible pre-selection of overly 'accepting' patients in the Waterworth and Luker study, there are clearly some patients who perceive nursing power as overwhelming, and as a result of this they accept or 'acquiesce'. To illustrate the notion of acquiescence in its most serious context I draw upon an informal conversation I had with Nick Masters who had metastatic cancer of the lung and which I detailed in my fieldnotes:

> Discussion with Nick Masters about the information he's had. He clearly feels 'towed along', however articulate he is, by the doctors' recommendations for deep X-ray therapy. He seems completely compliant. He talks about a "consultative model". He says he's not really been presented with different options. They've just told him what's best for him and he feels he's "just got to go along with it". He also offers his opinions about how he would be dealt with if he was awkward.

Nick was very aware of his position of vulnerability. He knew his diagnosis, but his previous experiences of challenging authority in hospitals had left him very cautious. He was prepared to negotiate on some issues, such as going home for the weekend, but had acquiesced to the medical view in the most important respect, his unpleasant, dangerous, and what proved to be ineffective treatment: deep X-rays.

145

Fineman (1991) gives examples of the strategies which clients are expected to adopt in accepting the treatment regime or plan. These include co-operating with the staff, being willing to follow reasonable suggestions, doing things in their own best interest, treating staff with respect and not presenting too many problems. Perhaps paradoxically, Fineman (p358) reports that "not say(ing) or do(ing) things just to please the staff" is also important. This seemed to be true in the case of the overly accepting Harold McGee whose total acquiescence was annoying to the staff, and through which he lost their respect.

Effective acquiescing then, in the context of social evaluation, was well judged; not too much and not too little; at least not from the staff's point of view. As others have argued (Lorber, 1975; Kelly and May, 1982) those aspects of client-professional interaction which make demands on the professional skills of the staff are likely to be highly valued. Seen as a skill, persuasion or the production of acquiescence in patients, is something to be valued for its own sake.

Whilst the literature relating to professional power in general and compliance in particular is very large, it is my intention here to draw attention only to the theoretical insights provided by a small number of very influential theorists. The discussion inevitably links heavily with that of clinical power as an aspect of the social climate in Howarth ward.

Avoiding stigma

First, I think it appropriate to discuss Goffman's (1968) view. Utilising his concept of 'moral career', it is possible to see how the patient's position is analogous to that of the inmate of a total institution. This is especially so in terms of the relationship between social identity or reputation and the behaviour of the staff. Much of the patient's behaviour can be explained in terms of the avoidance of a permanently deviant state or 'stigma'. Acquiescing is analogous to the process of learning the rules and recognising that failure to abide by the norm of submission will result in 'spoiled identity' or stigma.

Such thinking also has a relation to the notion of deviance within the labelling perspective of Lemert (1967). Lemert developed but did not originate the concepts of primary and secondary deviance. Primary deviance is taken to be the original problem, such as illness itself. Secondary deviance is that behaviour, including social roles associated with it, which arises as a result. Lemert argues that its main motivator is that secondary deviant behaviour is developed as a defence, attack or adaptation to the overt and covert problems created by people's reactions to the primary deviation.

It is easy to see how such models perhaps oversimplify reality. For example I could argue that if the patient's illness is classified as primary deviance, then acquiescence should be seen as secondary deviance. It is a strategy for managing social, in this case mainly nurses', reactions to the primary deviance or illness. Such a view is paradoxical however, since it seems to me that in all but the most extreme cases of the genre (such as Harold McGee), acquiescence is the normative behaviour expected by the nursing staff. Williams (1987) has argued that really secondary deviance amounts only to a permanent 'spoilage of identity'. An example would be the situation of the person with a psychiatric diagnosis for whom all behaviour is subsequently interpreted in that light. In such cases it is said that there is then amplification of deviance, that is the psychiatric behaviour becomes exaggerated. Such notions may have limited value in the relatively short term. However, long term patients like Harold McGee, the rather permanently acquiescent individual who had many hospital experiences may well have come to this state by such a route. Primary and secondary deviance as concepts may then have something to offer the analysis of the long term reputations people develop and live out in the social relations of hospital care.

Acquiescing: doing ward work

The Straussian (1982a) sociology of work perspective which has been useful in other areas of my analysis is also of some use here. Acquiescing means doing ward work, whether recognised as such or not. It means accepting the division of labour as it exists in that context. In some cases it will be observing the more ill patients and reporting their status to nursing staff. In others it means co-operating with painful or unpleasant procedures, enduring them with fortitude. It is with this focus that the concept of acquiescence has greatest moral impact, since it creates the conditions for morally dubious conduct, such as inflicting unnecessary and uncomfortable procedures without challenge.

An example was Jack Redford, an emaciated 67 year old man suffering from chest wall cancer which had spread. He had been bleeding from the rectum for days and had a number of transfusions. He looked cachectic and yet the surgeons were called to give an opinion upon his rectal bleeding. To do this they decided to subject Jack to a gastroscopic examination of the stomach and a sigmoidoscopy (to examine the colon). Although this seemed excessive in his condition the medical staff professed the opinion that if the bleeding was due to something less sinister than the malignancy, such as a polyp, they would not forgive themselves if he bled to death. Jack did not really want the procedures, but acquiesced when pressed by medical staff and his relatives, whose support they had recruited.

Perhaps in relation to this example it is appropriate to refer to the most abstract and yet possibly the most relevant theories explaining the context of acquiescence and its relation to social judgement.

Nurses: agents of medical control

In his paper on types of medical social control, Conrad (1979) shows the extent to which nurses can be conceived as being vicarious agents of medical control of deviance. He develops Freidson's (1970) thesis that nursing power derives almost wholly from association with a dominant professional group. The relevance of this, is that nurses' goals in achieving acquiescence with their aims for the client are but a first move in ensuring maximal compliance with medical regimes. By analogy, the nursing staff play the role of sergeant major by 'softening up' recruits through the strategy of, among others, humiliation. When people enter hospital it almost certainly in the knowledge that such strategies not only are available but that embarrassment, deprivation of privacy and abolition of key elements of individuality are the norm. Routines, wearing night clothes and relatively public scrutiny of taboo areas of life such as bowel habit are some examples to which I have referred earlier. So much is easily established even if one takes the view that this is not necessarily sinister, but merely a function of history and limited resources.

Producing 'docility'

It has however been argued that such discipline, such coercion as may exist within these social processes, is designed, through social evolution, to dissociate power from the body. It increases the aptitude of the body to produce labour, but diminishes it in terms of its power to resist exploitation. Acquiescence, which Foucault (1991) might term docility, is an aspect of the domination which those in power have over their subjects. Indeed he argues that power is diffuse but with a strong relationship to knowledge, especially scientific knowledge through which it is maintained. In a brief extract from his "Discipline and Punish" (1977) he suggests that a key factor in the production of 'docility' is the location of the individual in a constant state of surveillance which he names the Panopticon:

This enclosed, segmented space, observed at every point, in which the individuals are inserted in a fixed place, in which the slightest movements are supervised, in which all events are recorded, in which an uninterrupted work of writing links the centre and periphery, in which power is exercised without division, according to a continuous and hierarchical figure, in which each individual is constantly located, examined and distributed among the living beings, the sick and the dead - all this constitutes a compact model of the disciplinary mechanism. (p197)

This may be slightly overstated, but the description fits a medical ward even in the 1990s. All these features exist, indeed some the more so in recent times, such as the relatively detailed writing of the nursing process and the constant location of individuals by monitors or clear lines of visibility or audibility in wards designed for observation. Foucault presents a complex and polemical thesis, but which cannot fail to provoke important questions about the domination nurses and their allies the doctors have over peoples' bodies and their lives.

Conclusion

Acquiescing was a strategy for dealing with the difficulties faced by patients in the ward. It was sometimes the result of conflict of struggle, but not necessarily so. Some patients are aware of the strategy's importance as a means to a reasonable sociable reputation. Others are prepared to acquiesce only in certain respects as an aspect of negotiating. Clearly, however, acquiescing is an important part of complying with the wishes of the hospital staff. It can be seen as a process itself through which patients come to terms with compliance, and is part of the means through which patients allow nurses to consolidate and exercise power. I now intend to discuss some of the outcomes of nursing patients in a climate of social judgement. This involves strategies both for caring and for coping.

11 Aspects of caring and coping

I have thus far outlined some of the key features to be considered in a processual account of social judgement in the context I studied, a medical ward. Indeed my main in this book is to illuminate the process of social judgement from an interpretative perspective. At this point, I plan to discuss considerations arising out of the framework I have suggested. What follows is an account of selected strategies which we as nurses drew upon to manage care in the context of social judgement and some of our ways of dealing with the consequences. Aspects of caring and coping are inseparable in at least one important respect; that strategies for coping are often also ways of managing care and vice versa. I separate them within this chapter only for analytic and descriptive convenience. I will begin with a discussion of excellent care.

'Brilliant nursing'

It was clear that many nurses were aware that some patients were perceived as unpopular and others popular. As Neil (staff nurse) had hinted, nurses developed strategies to maintain standards of care in the face of patients being labelled as 'difficult' or 'demanding'. Some of these were initiated by individual nurses who were, like students Helen and Bill, keen to treat patients as they found them personally rather than as other nurses did. Others were led by experienced nurses as a matter of ward policy and would be explicitly or implicitly directed at preventing serious deterioration in care standards when patients were 'hard to nurse'. My discussion will focus upon some of these patients, with social evaluations of patients as a background against which the examples should be seen, rather than in each case a cause and effect relation being assumed.

I will discuss, as case studies, three situations in which the phenomenon which I typify as 'brilliant nursing' occurred. In my fieldwork and in my previous experiences I was aware that my occupational colleagues were aware of examples of highly skilled or devoted care. Rarely would this amount to care requiring technical skill. Rather, despite the widely acknowledged prestige and higher status of technical or intensive care nursing, brilliant care refers to detailed, well planned, and to some extent altruistic care. That is to say care that is above the routine requirements or the normative standards, and requires harder work or more personal discomfort than normal. I first learned of 'brilliant nursing' on an intensive care unit. I soon realised that I was most highly valued by my technically proficient colleagues not for my ability to diagnose cardiac arrhythmias but for my attention to much more basic matters, like the care of a person's mouth when it is invaded by rigid plastic tubing and a fungal infection, or scrupulously washing off electrode jelly after a diagnostic procedure.

At the time when Albert Littlewood's medical condition had deteriorated considerably, he became confused and very disorientated. He was clearly very ill from heart failure, but its sequelae of oxygen deprivation and body electrolyte imbalance were rendering his emotional state very aggressive. He was rarely lucid and yet was trying to get out of bed and was at risk of a fall. In my fieldnotes I document aspects of the ward report given to us that day by a staff nurse as we began a 1pm (late) shift:

Janice: Albert Littlewood, very confused, NFR (not for resuscitation). Probably a silent M.I. (myocardial infarction), restless, aggressive...No, violent! But he's weak, incontinent of urine. He's had three lots of haloperidol (sedative) and it hardly touched him...

We can see that it has been a struggle to provide adequate and safe care for Albert. A number of issues interested me from a moral point of view, such as the need for restraint and the fact that this patient had been most unpopular from the earliest day of his admission. But of relevance to my current point, I found that the nurse who had offered to 'special' him, that is to sit constantly by him to prevent him coming to harm, was the most senior nurse on the ward, the Sister. Indeed she had done this for much of the day. Whilst this was convenient in that it allowed Olivia, the third year finalist to practise ward management, it was no soft option. Being detailed to care for patients on a one-to one basis, is very demanding since it provides none of the usual opportunities for relief of tension available to those engaged in a co-operative effort. Given that on other occasions student nurses were sometimes critical of qualified staff being difficult to recruit into basic care, this action by the ward sister was symbolic. It showed her expectation of the role of experienced staff in relating directly to patients wherever possible. It seemed to me to make the statement to those present that "the care of this person is important despite our feelings about him as a person".

Another qualified nurse aware of the problem of unpopularity whilst acknowledging the nurses' need to moan was Neil. His view, not dissonant with my observations, was that he tried to do more for the patients he did not like. He had told me previously that in his experience patients often had an undisclosed reason for being 'unreasonable' so that whilst one might moan about them, one also had a responsibility to find out what the problem was. In the sense that such care was contrived and for people who did not seem likeable, this could have similarity with the concept of 'brilliant care'. In his own words:

Neil: From my point of view, if there's a patient on the side that I'm working on who is unpopular, I try to do more for that patient.The classic way of stopping a patient who buzzes every two minutes is to get there before he buzzes. And say "I've just come to see do you want anything only I'm going to do something else". And he'll say "No, no, I don't need anything" and stop buzzing.

This sort of approach to the management of 'attention-seeking' patients is documented by Bradby (1990) in her study of the status passage of British student nurses into the fully fledged occupational role. She notes that one of her older student informants had been surprised to learn that coping with demanding patients by 'being particularly helpful' had worked.

One day, I was able to spend some time getting to know the relatively unpopular Charles Eastwood, over whom Caroline and I had exchanged our 'knowing glances' but whom Neil assured me had another side to him. He may have been feeling a little better, but was able to talk between gasps for air as if this was now normal for him:

Long talk to Charles Eastwood. He perhaps sees himself as better educated than average (he's a graduate engineer) and is interested in my role. He seems impressed at my disclosure of my (usual) job and possession of a master's degree (both of which answers I cannot avoid without false modesty). He was really chatty, and we had quite a moving conversation about his experiences during the Second World War when he saw, from a Civil Defence Position (as a teenager), much of the Battle of Britain in 1940 and later on the loss of many American Bomber crews as they crashed in their badly damaged aircraft returning from raids. He comes across as rather right wing with some stereotyped attitudes to Asian patients on the ward, but, perhaps perceiving my discomfort (tactfully displayed I hope) tries to retrieve the situation with the more positive "they don't complain do they". This latter remark seemed meant to be a humorous comparison with his own behaviour into which he had more insight than I had imagined. It illustrated to me the possibilities for re-negotiation of personal evaluations through getting to know people.

Another example of care calculated to counteract the possible deleterious consequences of a 'difficult patient' label happened one afternoon. I have already described how it was that whilst Sam Read was on the whole popular or likeable, his highly dependent state as a result of his stroke and his complaints of genuine discomfort in a chair seemed to be irritating certain staff members. I too had found being responsible for his total care very hard work, especially as I was underconfident in my skills. In my notes, I recorded an incident of some complexity, and so I hope that I can, in mere text, give some indication of its meaning and its relation to my general argument. It involved Helen, the second year student nurse, and myself as mostly observer. The care was wholly initiated by Helen:

> After report Helen and I load Sam into bed with Janet's help. Once in and on his right side, Helen 'does his mouth' very diligently, and with a grace and humour I've not seen. She picks individual items of mince-meat out of his (half-paralysed) mouth and mops round it, encouraging him to exercise his tongue too, from side to side. I guess she's seen a speech therapist do this at the Rehab. Hospital, but she's still very patient and thoughtful. She chats him up and gets him smiling. When she asks him to show her his tongue, he's reluctant and suggests she do the same. She's a young woman, and the pseudo-sexual meaning behind this embarrasses her. (Perhaps because I'm there). She says "not likely" and he laughs too.

Writing up this note I could not help noting the subtlety, complexity and humanity of this moment. I knew that it had significance for my emerging view that the social judgement of people was based upon something rather more than lists of behavioural or diagnostic variables. It has also, if I have captured the moment at all, something to say about 'brilliant nursing', care which, in this example at least, combined recognition of a very disabled elderly man as someone with fundamental physical needs, and at least as important, a need for humour and personal interest.

It may be seen from my examples, that nursing of this type, 'brilliant nursing', has various features. It is not necessarily that which could be identified by an audit instrument. It depends, for its typification as such by ward nurses, upon their opinions of it being so. They will give

153

accounts of wards upon which they have worked where the nursing care was 'brilliant'. And they will not agree. For some the ideal is clearly prescribed and executed physical care. That, at least, is visible and recordable. For others it is exquisite understanding of patients' emotional needs. The concept is socially constructed. It has meaning for those who share in the culture of that time and that place and for others only insofar as it can be adequately described. I believe that for a time I was allowed some access to that culture, and that the concept had the meaning I have tried to illuminate with these examples. In any sense, these were some of the strategies employed by nurses in an attempt to mitigate the potential effects of unpopularity.

Doing the minimum: "nobody'll talk to them"

Sometimes however, mitigation did not obviously take place, and care was at a minimum level tolerable by nursing staff. Among my informants in the ward it was primarily student nurses who identified examples of patients receiving a lower standard of care from nursing staff than perhaps they might. Some students related this to the consensus ward view of the patient's worth, or popularity. As I will argue, despite a relatively relaxed atmosphere on the ward, the student nurses generally felt themselves to belong to a different status group to those who were qualified, and often had different perceptions. First year student Bill, who had studied some moral philosophy on a degree course, was aware that the moral problems he faced often were the "little things as well as the big issues". He had felt difficulties with deciding when, to whom, and how much time to allocate to talking to patients on the ward. He felt that allocation of resources such as nursing time was an important issue, and made it clear that the allocation was not always as he would wish it:

Bill: There's always just the little things as well as the big issues. Every day you come on the ward, there's little things like talking to somebody, not talking to somebody, choosing which patient to do before another.

Helen, a student in her second year echoed Bill's view, and emphasised that often decisions about care were related to the ward view of the patient:

Helen: Well it's so important but when a patient is demanding basically nobody'll sit down and actually talk to them, like they'll talk to others that aren't so demanding. Really they should get as much nursing time as the others. There are definitely patients people talk to and ones they don't. That's so important I think.

Helen's view was that sometimes patients could re-negotiate their position, perhaps by being less demanding of nurses' attention. This she felt sometimes happened as a natural consequence of improved physical well-being, which left the paradoxical situation she describes here in relation to Jimmy Mackindoe, a recovering stroke patient:

Helen: But then he's better now so his manner's more pleasant and he's more skilled at getting things in a roundabout way. And suddenly everyone thinks he's O.K. But that's just because he's a bit better, so the poorly patient didn't get the care and now he's a bit better he's getting better treatment. And that's wrong.

Most of the time, both in fieldwork and in interviews, I gained the impression that where unpopular patients did receive less diligent care, it was in the interpersonal dimension. That is to say that nurses rarely avoided giving physical care. Indeed the need for physical care is usually clear and explicit, and its absence is more easily noticed. Nurses are, and feel, more easily accountable for the physical care they give than the psychological care they may be able to provide. An increasing literature details the low priority given by nurses to psychological care of patients. Various studies have provided evidence that nurses interact most with those who can initiate conversations themselves, and that even in the provision of comprehensive physical care they may have very little purposive interaction with their patient (Stockwell, 1972; Fielding, 1986).

My third year student colleague, Susan, was able to explain briefly how she saw the management of unpopularity, at least in respect of the physical care of Albert Littlewood. He, as I have described, was becoming extremely difficult to manage both physically and interpersonally:

Susan: But I mean, it must have changed because otherwise nobody would have been prepared to sit there and give him his dinner.

Compensating for labels

Knowing that patients were seen as good or bad, popular or unpopular was a source of concern to most, if not all, of the nurses in Howarth ward. I have referred to various strategies through which individual staff attempted to ameliorate any negative consequences of such an evaluation.

Nicky James (1989) draws upon Strauss's (1982b) concepts of 'comfort work' and 'composure work' to show how nursing staff do their best to ameliorate the emotional and physical discomforts of illness and its treatment. I have shown how sometimes nurses both overtly and covertly performed excellent care, with exquisite attention to detail and in full consideration of the emotional needs of patients. They called this 'brilliant nursing', a phrase which though not universal, was used at a conference by Richard Wells to describe the excellent care he had received during a relapse due to Acquired Immune Deficiency Syndrome (Nursing Times, 1992). He died in January 1993.

Bradby (1990) describes how nurses saw 'being especially helpful' as a way of coping with the stresses and strains of nursing the patients whose demands were very exacting, and of coping with stigmata with which patients were associated. She notes the difficulties posed by trying to behave 'as if the stigma doesn't exist', such as where patients had stomas which caused some nurses to feel 'sickened'. These responses Bradby (1990) describes as 'adaptive', and they can be seen to be an attempt to normalise relations in these circumstances.

Carl May (1992) analyses staff nurses' attempts to 'know about' their patients and the problems which arise in so doing. Acknowledging a theoretical allegiance to Michel Foucault, May attempts to show how nurses did their best to ameliorate the negative effects of reductive medical knowledge. By this he seems to mean that the nurses sought to know their patients more comprehensively than simply in terms of "more or less problematic pathological categories" (p483). May implies that such strategies of more holistic 'knowing' are ways of compensating for the inadequacies of the medical approach. However, from a truly Foucauldian perspective this knowing or in Foucault's terms 'surveillance' may be just as disempowering for clients.

In her ethnographic study of a casualty department which continued the long tradition of such studies, Helen Roberts (1992) is at pains to point out that people labelled as 'rubbish' were not necessarily treated as such. In her afternotes to this paper she develops the point that in other studies (in the USA) severely handicapped neonates were sometimes referred to as 'premie trash' and 'trainwrecks'. She suggests that this terminology is not meant to be heard by parents or outsiders, and the assumption is that these labels only act as a venting of the nurses' frustration and do not affect the standard of care. Roberts goes on, however, to note that those with an interest in the power of naming would not dismiss the possible negative consequences so lightly.

If however, despite an expressed negative social judgement, patients are treated by staff as well as or better than should be expected, then this could be said to be an aspect of compensating for the label. Compensating seems also to be an aspect of what has increasingly been referred to as patient advocacy. Christine Webb (1987) reviews various definitions of advocacy concluding that informing the client and giving support in whatever decisions are arrived at are the most important facets of the advocate role. Webb suggests a number of the strategies which nurses may adopt in acting as an advocate for a patient. These include giving information, ensuring that treatments and other activities are properly explained and if necessary complaining about inappropriate care or treatment. Of course, she is sensitive to the difficulties posed by the role of advocate in the health care context within a framework of medical and managerial domination of the occupation of nursing. A number of precedents have caused British nurses to be cautious about being too public in their advocacy (Beardshaw, 1981), especially when, as Webb argues, they often lack the confidence, assertiveness and negotiation skills necessary for a satisfactory outcome for all concerned.

Whilst Webb alludes in her discussion of her advocate role to giving information to her respondents during a major research project, most discussion of advocacy has been of its more public or overt variety. My category of 'brilliant nursing' was, I will argue, often a covert form of advocacy. By taking special care to compensate for a negative social judgement nurses in general, and student nurses in particular, were acting as patient advocates, but in a covert way. Their excellent practice was often an attempt to subvert what they saw as the potential consequences of a negative social judgement which had been expressed and was perhaps common currency in the ward report. I have referred previously to Melia's (1984) use of the concept of segmentation to mean that the students have two sets of expectations to meet. I would argue that, in respect of compensating, nurses who chose to give 'brilliant care' covertly were using a similar strategy to separate their public ward image and values from those they expressed privately to patients and friends.

It is impossible to escape the clear link between such a strategy and its consequences for the nursing staff in terms of anxiety. I will consequently outline some aspects of nurses' 'coping' later in this chapter. Next however, I wish to discuss some aspects of paternalism.

Stepping in

It might seem that 'stepping in' is a contrast to the other strategies I describe. This may be an oversimplification. Rather, stepping in is the way in which nurses act, believing their actions to be in the best interests of their patients. Sometimes such actions, well justified paternalism if you will, are 'brilliant nursing' by the nurses' definition. Sometimes this would be less easily argued. An illustration of the fine balance or mixture of approaches may become evident if I continue to describe the care of Albert Littlewood who was very ill from heart failure and who had become violent and aggressive. I have noted that nursing staff were prepared to sit constantly by him to monitor him and if necessary prevent accidents such as a fall. He was in a side ward by now, partly because he was embarrassing patients and relatives in the ward by throwing his bedcovers off and getting naked out of the bed. One staff nurse, Elaine, was very frustrated by his behaviour, and gave those of us coming on a late shift an indication of the tactics she had employed in managing his care over the previous two shifts which I summarised in my fieldnotes:

Elaine: He throws the covers off and he's naked. His relatives came in and he was naked and uncovered behind the screens, and she (his wife) was upset, I don't think she realised how he is, we've done our best to keep him covered and clothed.

I could see for myself that there was evidence that he had been tied by a linen sheet and Elaine discussed the nurses' attempts to restrain Albert in the bed with sheets and blankets. The cot sides were inadequate to this sort of purpose and would only prevent people rolling out of a bed. Elaine also mentioned her tactics in ensuring that Albert received sedation:

Elaine: He spits it out, we even gave it to him in strawberry jam yesterday, till he realised and spat it out, almost in my face, I was too smug.

In this example a number of points emerge about Elaine's plan of care for Albert Littlewood. Whilst some of the nurses are prepared to sit with him for long periods, this is seen as a thankless and difficult duty. She has therefore tried to ensure Albert's safety, and her own peace of mind, by using coercive measures. First, the restraint within the bed by means of sheets and blankets carefully tied and tucked in, and second by trying to give him sedation camouflaged in jam.

Such tactics should be debated at length. It could be argued that Albert's interests were indeed the primary concern of these nurses, that is they were trying to prevent both injury and indignity from his getting out of bed in such a confused state. On the other hand these devices may have merely been expedient attempts to reduce nursing time spent 'specialling' Albert, and to reduce the chance of legal proceedings should he be injured falling out of bed, for which the nurses would surely be held responsible.

The measure that were used here do seem open to criticism if we take the view that patients have a right to informed consent before being given medication and a right not to be restrained except under the terms of an order under the relevant Mental Health Act for their own protection (not the case here). If, in discussing this case I seem a little judgemental of the nurses' actions, I too faced moral dilemmas in my management of care the justification for which still gives me cause for concern.

Sam Read had recovered consciousness after a very severe stroke but was still completely paralysed down his left side and was very heavy. Earlier I described how Helen cleaned his mouth after lunch. I find in my fieldnotes a stark example of what can only be described as my coercion of Sam, who could hardly have been more vulnerable. I had been working on Sam's side of the ward during my days there and had come to admire his honesty and stoicism. I also found caring for him very challenging because it tested all of my basic skills. I still had them, but lacked confidence from having increasingly worked as a classroom teacher rather than a clinician. I will relate the incident in full from my notes made at the time:

Sam's constipated and has had enemas before with minimal result. His oral aperients don't seem to work, so a phosphate enema was suggested to me in the ward report. It needs to be 'written up' these days, so we bleeped the house officer. By 11.15 am finally the enema was prescribed so I got first year student Paula to help and we talked to Sam about it. Of course he didn't like the idea. "It'll just leave me in a pool of diarrhoea in the bed 'cos I won't be able to hold it," he said. "Anyway it'll hurt 'cos I've got piles. I don't need it, just let me sit on the toilet for an hour or two," he argued. I decided to try with my 'caring sympathetic' voice (and conscious of Paula watching my every move) to explain how he's too ill to sit there on the toilet for a few minutes let alone two hours (He can't support himself in an armchair). Although I can see that Paula isn't troubled by my persuasion, I am, and finally say to Sam "There's not much choice". Again he complains that the probable mess in the bed will be embarrassing and I feel even worse.

I put the jelly on the enema tip, put a glove on a gently insert the catheter. He yelps (the piles I suppose) but soon settles. I ask him to try to keep it in and Paula kneels down to see if she can hold a pad under him in case of leakage and to stop us being sprayed if the fluid returns under pressure. Just then a rush of gas close to Paula embarrasses us all--but she never flinches. At least what's left of his dignity is preserved by her silence. A bit of brown fluid leaks and Sam's worried he'll mess the bed. I ask him to hold on and amazingly he does so. I leave the tube in acting as a plug for what seems like five minutes and it seems to work. Then Paula and I recruit Olivia to the task of getting him out of bed and on to the commode. I'm behind his head, Paula on the legs, and Olivia takes the weight of his bottom with it's attendant risk of leakage. Under her breath and always the wit, she muses "I guess I drew the short straw", but I can tell she's just amused, not disgusted.

We manage to get him on to the commode and with support he sits patiently making appropriate noises and smells. I've not felt so bad about a 'success' in a long while.

The more I think about this the more I know that I coerced rather than persuaded Sam to allow me to give him the enema. The pressures on me to do so were considerable. I had been asked to do the enema by the nurse in charge. Sam was visibly constipated. He drank little and had difficulty eating a bit of mince let alone a balanced high fibre diet. Other medications such as lactulose had also produced no result. I was still trying to show that at least in the area of this sort of care I was willing and keen to do my bit. Avoiding such a 'dirty job' would, I felt, have been seen as a serious weakness in my claim to be a real participant in the ward action. Wolf (1988) observes that " if an R.N. (qualified nurse) earned the reputation of consistently avoiding excreta, she was seen in a negative light" (p209). The enema was, after all, just part of the care that we gave to Sam that day, and it was of course sensible to allow him a bath afterwards which we did. I knew that if I found some excuse not to do it, someone else would give it.

Since the claims that nurses have been making to the provision of more individualised care than in the past, it may be more likely that in such matters many patients would have more power to refuse a remedy for constipation, or for that matter a remedy for anything. I will argue, however, that such powers are still seriously limited in respect of medical treatments (i.e. those prescribed by doctors). In the case of nursing prescriptions clients or patients may be achieving a modest empowerment in certain areas of care, as much because assessment of needs is arguably more detailed than it was, and because some routinisation has been reduced. Technically the enema was medically prescribed, but it was given wholly upon the assessment and planning advice of nurses, and so I suggest that it was a nursing prescription.

Sam Read, however, was disempowered in relation to this particular aspect of his physical and emotional needs. I, therefore, was empowered to decide his needs, and to infringe his personal liberty in a very intimate, and to some extent public way. He protested a little. I ask myself how much he would have had to protest before I would have recognised a right for Sam to decide for himself, even if he was wrong on clinical grounds. In particular, and related to my general point in this chapter, what moral or social judgement of Sam caused me to limit his autonomy in a way which I might not have done with some other individual?

160

Jenny Littlewood (1991) makes lucid observations upon the role of the nurse in the encouragement of compliance, using in particular the example of body waste management to make her point:

> Nurses become intimately involved and identified with the containment of personal pollution. A sick person has undergone several changes - having changed from obeying rules of when to eliminate, eat or move about according to an accepted social role of being sick and out of control. The sick person has transgressed social rules, has disobeyed accepted ideas on behaviour in space and time. (Littlewood,1991:178)

Littlewood identifies the nature of communication about 'bowels' between nurses and patients as a means of persuasion, a means of asserting authority which should result in compliance in other matters:

> It is a means of persuasion...disruption of bowel function is one of the earliest bodily signs of distress and can produce signs of psychological distress. It is also the focus of an early attempt to control behaviour... The patient must 'behave' in order to be healed. (Littlewood, 1991:181)

Littlewood's suggestion is that, as with other aspects of health care, nurses use the patients' 'illness' as legitimation for their control of their patients' bodily functions. As she puts it, nurses use humiliation as a tactic for control, a control the medical staff need in order to focus down upon the disease rather than be too concerned for the whole person. According to this view, I was, in coercing Sam to have the enema, engaging in a symbolic act of disempowerment, one calculated to further the cause of compliance with medical and nursing plans. This insight into the social processes used in engaging compliance was commented upon by third year student Louise:

Louise: It seems to be that you get into the kind of mode of working in the place and you don't question as much as you did before. And it's true that when they're in hospital you don't ask, you say you've got to do this for them, you've got to do that, you don't normally ask them what they want. It's all too easy as a nurse in uniform to persuade people to do something.

Paternalism

The idea of paternalism (to use the patriarchal term rather than maternalism) of knowing what is best for recipients of health care, is broadly inconsistent with the notion of individualised care. In my observations and in the interviews some nurses were keen to point out the degree to which they felt patients were consulted about their care. It was as if consultation established an area of control for patients but which did not amount to real autonomy. Even those patients deemed to be self-caring, that is able to bathe themselves without help, were likely to be subjected to persuasion once a certain point was reached. Staff nurse Rachel seemed to feel that some patients saw it as part of the patient role to resist the nurses' wish that they were bathed:

Rachel: If someone doesn't want a bath I feel comfortable with it. But then again there are some patients who say "No, no, no, no, never." And then I think you have to step in for their sake, and for everyone else's sake. To stop them being smelly.

Here she seems to locate their resistance more in game being played by patients to test nurses' resolve than in any real perception of patient autonomy. Littlewood's (1991) parallel with a mother and child relationship is helpful here if indeed patients are playing games and not trying to maintain their individuality. Rachel goes on to identify a slightly different notion, that of patients wanting and expecting to be 'pushed' by nurses.

Rachel: But some people will take on the sick role and they want you to step in and push a bit to try and keep them as independent as possible. Or else they become poorly.

Rachel seems to feel that much of the legitimation for 'stepping in' arises from patients' expectations of the nurse patient relationship. That patients expect and behave as if the nurses possess legitimate authority. In the American context Wolf (1988) finds similarly:

Nurses on the day shift insisted that able patients "get washed up now". Their insistence was hard to ignore. Even the most bath resistant patients usually complied. (Wolf, 1988:185)

Again Littlewood's notion of the nurse behaving as a 'concerned mother' suggests some agreed legitimation of this situation in context. Littlewood's discussion is explicitly from a feminist perspective, and she chooses to make her parallels between patients and children, and nurses and mothers. Therefore it seems worthwhile briefly to explore the use of terms like 'maternalism' rather than 'paternalism' in this context. Benjamin and Curtis (1981) argue that the gender neutral term 'parentalism' should be used in such discussions. They continue to define this supposedly neutral term in the fashion of paternalism, that is, 'father knows best' or as Geddie (1964) suggests, 'unwelcome interference'. It seems to me that this device is self defeating. This use of parentalism implies that women have equal power in our society to determine the needs and wants of others. Though not so widely used, the idea of maternalism is not the same and so the half way term, parentalism, does not satisfactorily make a bridge here. Maternalism has a more benevolent meaning, one of nurturance, care and support.

Stepping in: "we're going to keep him here now"

In the fieldwork I came across and was involved in many examples of the management of care by means of 'stepping in', or disempowering patients. As I note earlier, Rachel had used this term to illustrate why she insisted on bathing patients that she felt were becoming smelly. I will discuss one further instance here, notable because it related to a patient who had become in many ways physically independent of nursing staff after a period of grave illness and considerable dependence.

Robert Munro was a recovering homeless alcoholic who also had tuberculosis. At a later point in my fieldwork, he was well enough to walk around the ward, to bathe himself when encouraged to do so, and could have left the hospital had he chosen to do so and had he been allowed to. I shared the predictions of medical and nursing staff that if he did leave he would probably succumb to untreated tuberculosis, malnutrition or pneumonia. Being homeless in his weakened and recently very ill state was a grave risk. Drinking heavily, also fairly predictable without other social supports would speed this process.

As one tactic to avoid his leaving, Robert was not allowed to have his outdoor clothes. This tactic is also used in psychiatric units when individuals are to be discouraged from leaving or are detained against their will on a Section of the Mental Health Act. Robert was not legally detained under a section of this Act. He was, however, detained. Much of the time Robert seemed to accept his need for hospital or other support, to recover from illness and to avoid drinking. Some of the nurses were troubled by the problem. Third year student Louise put it this way:

Louise: He's another case I feel strongly about, I realise that for his health's sake it would be better for him to have his medication, and also for the sake of other people outside, who he could pass his T.B. (tuberculosis) on to. But on the other hand I find it absolutely appalling that people (doctors) can come on the ward and say, "We'll keep him sedated so that he

163

doesn't leave the hospital, as he'll not continue his therapy". I mean, who are we to say to anybody "You've got no choice, you've got to stay here". That's what's so wrong, the reason they won't give him his clothes is because they think he'll leave.

Louise could see the rationale, but seemed to feel that Robert's co-operation with the policy was not sought in discussion with him. According to my reading of the situation, Robert on some days would see the importance, to him, of getting better. On other days the strategy for achieving this goal, complying with treatment, seemed inconsistent with his previous lifestyle. This particular problem became a focus of my informants' attention in a number of interviews. Most of the nurses could see the dilemma, that satisfying their own goals of cure and compliance meant limiting Robert's autonomy. The justification offered was that on good days Robert could see the sense of the policy in his own and others' interests. This fact allowed his detention on bad days until he recovered his composure and understanding of the benefits of treatment.

The context of these strategies for managing care is, as I have tried to show, one in which patients are socially and morally judged by nurses. Robert Munro was quite disliked by many. If common sense has any value, it would have said that nurses would have seen his life as less worthwhile than others, particularly as some of his own behaviours devalued the worth of his life in their eyes. That they went to such lengths to preserve his life against a background of grave uncertainty about his future and his own wish to change to a more survivable lifestyle is interesting. It shows the dominance that preservation of life has as an ideology irrespective of predictors of success.

'Stepping in' is widespread in the management of care. To some extent some thought is given to the notion of individual autonomy, but in many cases nurses will override autonomy in what they claim to be client interest. Many of my informants were aware of this and saw it as a problem. However they felt that the social fabric, the social structures within which they operated did not easily allow alternatives to 'stepping in'.

Coping in a context of social judgement

In this section I intend to give an account of some of the chief coping strategies which emerged during my fieldwork. It is important to remember that separation between categories is really only a convenience, for analytic purposes. Perhaps a key example is the way in which 'grumbling' about patients is both a mode of construction of judgemental

164

evaluations of the patients *and* a coping strategy for nurses faced sometimes with the profound demands of both physical an emotional labour.

Nurses: "going along"

On one occasion I was able to chat openly and informally with two third year student nurses on the ward, one of whom I was able to interview in greater depth later. Louise, the most vocal, was interested in my focus upon the moral problems that nurses face each day. She was quick to observe, however, that often these issues are not very evident when you are busy and involved in a practical way in what is going on. My approximately verbatim record of her remarks is:

Louise: You accept routine ways of doing things, you become socialised. Without deliberately conforming to be accepted you actually do just go along to get through the day.

Louise seems to be saying that 'going along' with things was not a deliberate strategy. but one that was an inevitable part of the routine for survival from day to day. To some extent nurses were pre-occupied with practical matters often of some urgency, which precluded deep thought about the moral difficulties which might be present. Also implied was that this conformity was to what the qualified nurses deemed to be appropriate. Olivia, an extrovert third year student nurse who did seem able to relate well to the qualified nurses, was also aware of the power the staff nurses had to make life difficult for a student with whom they did not see eye to eye:

Olivia: ...there was a staff nurse that didn't think that Bill (first year) was pulling his weight, and I worked with him loads of times and thought he was exceptional for the stage of training he was in. You find yourself trying to criticise them (students) 'cos somebody else in the senior grade criticises them. You think there must be something wrong.

Here I believe we see two social processes. First there is the power of the staff nurses to define good and bad students. Second, Olivia draws attention to the sanction of criticism, from which it is hard to dissent. Melia (1987) discusses the pressure put on students to be seen as 'pulling their weight', and to the fact that they would engage in spurious 'looking busy' behaviour rather than talk to patients, which was not 'getting through the work'. Whilst it was evident to me in my field work that talking to patients was a much more acceptable activity for students to undertake than Melia found, it was much more likely to occur in an afternoon when much of the hygiene care or 'horsework' had been done. I was able to explore this theme with Bill, whom Olivia had perceived as at risk of criticism from a staff nurse. Though still a relative neophyte, he had a deep understanding of the social and historical context in which he was operating:

Bill:　　　I find myself in a situation where I'm toeing the line, I might think about it (a moral dilemma) and discuss it afterwards, but in a situation with someone else I don't honestly go against what the staff nurses want.

Bill's view seemed to be that in his early days as a student compliance with ward policy was the best way to survive. He had a clear view of the possible consequences of serious public dissent and seemed to be saying that until he had more formal authority there was little to be gained from being deviant:

Bill:　　　I think perhaps nursing is all about custom and tradition, and do what was done before, it's not necessarily the correct way of doing something but it's done within the UKCC Code of Practice (Conduct) even though it may not be suitable morally to you.

Here Bill was referring to wider pressure than the interpersonal sanctions that Olivia had mentioned. He was clearly aware of a well known case in which a staff nurse had been suspended and disciplined consequent upon complaints he had made to his Health Authority and then the newspapers about poor staffing levels in a care of the elderly area:

Bill:　　　Being employed by a Health Authority or a Trust, nurses are open to conflict between employment by the Health Authority and the Code of Conduct. They could blow the whistle and end up losing their jobs and things like that.

This most thoughtful of respondents was clearly aware of the dangers of not 'toeing the line'. He was, however, still one of the nurses who seemed to make an effort to spend time with those patients who were unpopular with the other nurses. So he was aware of the tightrope he was walking when he did this, but felt that there were even more serious issues that he could not confront in the prevailing climate. As Melia describes it:

The 'fitting in' behaviour described by the students...supports the notion that students temporarily abandon their long-term, altruistic, professional-type goals in favour of meeting the requirements of the moment. (Melia, 1987: 169)

This view, that occupational socialisation is far from the permanent instillation of consistent values grew out of Becker et. al.'s (1961) interpretative study of medical student socialisation. In that study Becker argues that social behaviour and attitudes are contextual, that is they arise out of negotiation between the parties involved. In the context I describe, students such as Bill were expressing their own personal values in their work, but usually only insofar as they were not liable to intolerable sanctions.

"Keeping your head down"

Other students also referred to 'keeping their heads down' as a survival strategy. Some had experimented with putting their views across on controversial matters but had learned that it was usually not worth it. I asked third year Louise whether she thought that ward progress reports (continuous assessment of practice) had a part to play in encouraging compliant behaviour among students:

Louise: No, I don't think so... I think it's more like, just like a psychological sanction really. I've heard how students nurses have been discussed in derogatory terms, in a kind of official capacity. So you feel that "I don't want them saying that about me."

Louise was, by definition, relatively successful. That is, she had got through most of her training. She seemed to feel that ward progress reports were not very important, but the more junior students were less assured in this respect. They saw the assessment process and its accompanying written record as a threat. One such was Theresa, who gave me an account of an occasion when she had tried to act as an advocate for a female patient on another ward, and had paid a price:

Theresa: I'd seen an auxiliary nurse shout at a patient to get up. She really did say "...now come on stop messing this student nurse about," and the patient started crying and I felt obliged to stick up for the patient. I swear all I said was "actually I helped her this morning, she's just fallen over you know."

Theresa told me how a staff nurse who had not seen this incident nevertheless mentioned it in her final ward report, from which Theresa then knew that the auxiliary and the staff nurse had discussed it behind her back. She said that even the remark "needs to be more tactful and diplomatic" which the staff nurse had made was geared much more to the auxiliary's feelings than those of the patient who had been so upset at the time. Theresa suggested that on subsequent occasions she had felt guilty about 'keeping her head down'. On another occasion she had gone home feeling quite cowardly because she had failed to 'stick up for' another patient who was being coerced to eat some food he clearly did not want:

Theresa: I just keep my head down really but I thought afterwards that was really quite cowardly, I should have stuck up for him and there's been many instances where I've thought that's it, 'the unpopular patient'.

It seems then, that once they had learned the 'unwritten rules' as Melia (1987) terms them, junior students tended to be quite deferential toward their qualified colleagues. Even the more experienced third years were cautious in making their opinions known. Anita summed up the approach she would feel she had to take like this:

Anita: I'd start by going to what I thought was a sympathetic staff nurse, and I'd tend to ask them questions to try to get them thinking. A 'why are we doing this' sort of approach. And find out what their answer is and then get it into more of an argument about the pros and cons of something afterwards.

Later she suggested that this approach avoided criticism because all one was really doing was asking for clarification. The approach was 'polite'. It made sure that the staff nurse could clear up any misunderstood facts before the debate began. Seeking information was not the same as challenging expertise or authority. Leonard Stein (1978) outlined an analogous process in the relationship between doctors and nurses, in which nurses proffer advice but in a way in which the doctor does not lose face. Pembrey (1979) has similarly argued that as a result of the higher status of the medical staff in hospitals, ward sisters use various tactics to get the doctors to accept their advice. These tactics arise out of the socialised inferiority of the nursing staff, and are characterised by deference, flirtation and stealth. By this she means that various lifeskills are necessary to overcome the inherent imbalance in legitimate authority to determine treatment and care. Whilst the authority of the more senior nurses to determine policy is quite reasonably based upon their

168

qualification and their experience, students are forced to resort to skills of negotiation analogous to those Pembrey and Stein describe. That is, the skills of negotiating from a position of weakness.

The student nurses I worked with and spoke to did not seem particularly unhappy. Indeed they saw the ward as more than usually relaxed. The overall context, however, is one in which they have a definite conception of their lowly place in the hospital and ward hierarchy. This conception is maintained by their relative vulnerability on several grounds. They are subject to review by qualified staff in the normal course of their progress reports. They are aware that the qualified staff form an opinion about them which, they feel, can be based upon an unrepresentative aspect of their behaviour. Students did feel that a number of symbolic actions conferred status. Not least of these was 'being in the office', which, apart from at specific invited times, was not their province. Indeed even experienced students noted that one of the problems with caring for the heavier patients was that you had to "get them out of the office" to help you. Melia's (1987) distinction between 'us and them' was certainly evident.

Social distance

It would be easy to document this situation and imply that this is necessarily wrong. Popular theory of adult education would suggest that "hierarchical status boundaries and division of labour ought to be challenged and broken down" (Knowles, 1978).

Some thought, however, has to be given to the use of social distance as a means of managing the role of nurse, whether that of student or staff nurse. The influential work by Menzies (1960) is often cited, it seems to me, in support of this drive to humanise relationships by breaking down boundaries between staff of different roles and between staff and patients. Menzies, a psychoanalyst herself, draws from her data the conclusion that social distance and routines are used to defend the staff against anxieties inherent in their work. This conclusion, even given the complexity of theory from which she reasons, is reasonable. To conclude even further, that such rituals and boundaries must be removed seems to me to go beyond the data. Menzies provided no evidence for the superiority of a system which had removed these boundaries and Melia (1987) hypothesises tentatively that students disliked individualised care because some of the protection from anxiety is removed.

The examples I have given support a view that student nurses still conceive of themselves as of very low status in the ward and hospital pecking order. On the whole they comply with the dominant view of treatment and care promulgated by qualified nurses, and have to be very deferential and tactful in negotiating differing aims of care on the rare occasions that they do this. This seems to be so despite the evidence I provide that in many cases students are acutely aware of moral difficulties in the work they are asked to do and the treatment and care they are asked to provide. I was aware that many of my student informants had been hurt in learning these 'unwritten rules' by trial and error, by transgressing the norms and having sanctions applied. In these circumstances it seems naive to assume, except in the most extreme of circumstances, that students can act as advocates for patients' views in an effective way.

I have focused in particular upon the students because it was in their case that conformity to ward norms was most troubling to me. Naturally the less experienced or less assertive staff nurses also occasionally had difficulties putting their view across, but this did not seem so easily explained by an artificially constructed definition of role and status.

Feeling guilty

Working in this context led some nurses to experience guilt feelings about the way they labelled patients. The experienced staff nurse, Catherine, had got rather annoyed on one occasion with a patient:

Catherine: Actually I do think it's quite bad. I was quite conscious of it today when I was handing over, and I would say these things about him, and think, "well that's bad really".

MJ: How do we distinguish between appropriate professional communication and value judgements?

Catherine: I think nurses have to be very careful, I think I was guilty, like today, of labelling him, because I got so cross basically. And it's not very good really.

MJ: I think I know why you feel that way...

Catherine: But you've got to grumble, 'cos you've got to let your own feeling out. If you've had to put up with someone's unreasonable behaviour, you've got to get some of the frustration out. You can't do it with the patient, so the only way you've got to do it is with the nurses.

Of equivalent if not greater import was the feeling that some nurses had that they 'should have stuck up' for patients when they were being labelled negatively by others. Despite these feelings, students and the less experienced staff nurses learned to 'keep their heads down', because the sanction of becoming unpopular themselves was too hard to bear. Students generally learned to know their place, an observation in common with Buckenham and McGrath (1983). As Melia (1987) shows, students learn that they are just passing through and so to challenge orthodoxy openly is unwise. In the ward context, students 'fit in' for the most part and go along with the ethos they find. Occasionally students would find themselves able to challenge the dominant view of a patient, but this could only be done in the quiet confidence of already having established a good reputation with the senior staff. Second year student Helen seemed able to do this to some degree, since she employed considerable maturity and social skill in all her relations with both staff and patients. Others more 'green' would soon learn that 'toeing the line' was safer for the time being.

Luker (1984), whilst discussing the deviance of being a degree student of nursing (then a relative rarity), draws upon the sociology of stigma to explain how these students manage their difference. They first adopt a strategy of normalisation analogous to 'keeping their head down'. Later as they develop confidence in their knowledge base and come to appreciate the advantages as well as the difficulties posed by their differentness, some are able to branch out, as it were, and appear to be more overtly different. Equally, both staff and students seemed to need to establish a secure base from which eventually to challenge orthodox views.

Strategic compliance

In a study of the occupational socialisation of social workers, Rosaline Barbour (1985) discusses the concepts of 'strategic compliance' and 'internalised adjustment' which seem to summarise these processes. The former is the individual complying with the definition of the situation rendered by those in authority and accepting the constraints of their situation, whilst maintaining private reservations. Internalised adjustment is when the individual not only complies but believes that the constraints they are under (such as agreeing with an evaluative label) are for the best. Barbour does not use these ideas uncritically, and is herself concerned that they may offer only impressionistic guidelines for empirical study of differing patterns of occupational socialisation. Interestingly she too draws upon Goffman's (1968) concept of 'moral career'. This, she argues is more useful since it typifies an individual's position as sequential and negotiable rather than permanent in the sense that the previous categories imply. This notion seems useful in analysing the coping strategies that nurses use in the context of social judgement because it would be wrong to imply that nurses fall neatly into categories. Rather they adopt different strategies for compliance, or indeed dissidence, as they perceive is appropriate and consistent with their 'occupational survival'.

Turner (1987) suggests that a key strategy through which nurses (at a certain level) maintain solidarity in the face of an institutional hierarchy is complaint. He argues that complaining is a crucial feature of occupational subcultures where solidarity is an important aspect of resistance. Of course much of this complaint is directed at those perceived to be in authority, but there is no doubt that off-stage complaints about patients are also a key coping strategy even if this means that they are also the origin of judgemental evaluations of patients. An issue here is whether ward reports ought to be seen as off-stage for this purpose, and whether it is useful to distinguish between physical locations in which social judgements of this type are made.

Strauss and Glaser (1964) drew early attention to the way in which nurses avoided patients whom they knew to be dying. Other studies have revealed similar phenomena when nurses are presented with emotionally or even physically challenging situations (Smith, 1992). It could be argued that the routinisation, task-orientation and splitting of the nurse-patient relationship described by Menzies (1960) was an institutionalised avoidance of emotional closeness with patients. Indeed Menzies herself saw these as tactics constructed as defences against the inherent anxiety of nurse-patient relations in hospitals.

The professional prescriptive literature (see for example Kershaw and Salvage, 1986 or Aggleton and Chalmers, 1986) continues mainly to urge adoption of 'patient centred' approaches to care. Relatively little attention has, however, been devoted to the need for avoidance as a legitimate coping mechanism. Indeed some forms of overt avoidance behaviour are labelled absenteeism (mostly students) or burn-out (highly-qualified staff). That is to say, avoidance is not constructed as a legitimate coping strategy.

Conclusion

In this chapter I have analysed some principal features of the way that nursing care is managed in the context of social judgement and ways in which nurses on the ward cope with the difficult moral milieu in which they live and work.

Sometimes we pay less attention, in the interpersonal dimension at least, to those we consider to be unpopular. More commonly, however, according to my observations where patients might possibly be seen as undeserving, strategies are utilised to ensure that a high standard of care is maintained. One of these is the giving of 'brilliant care'. This can be either directed by the senior nurses, or if necessary is practiced covertly by more junior nurses who do not feel that they ought to challenge the official negative view of a patient. Another vitally important strategy for managing care in the ward was paternalism, in the form of stepping in, a term commonly used by my respondents. Stepping in was necessarily based upon a judgement of the right to autonomy of the individual patient, and therefore had a good deal to do with the social evaluation which had taken place. Since these strategies were rarely applied through a consensus of opinion of the nursing staff or indeed their patients, they had the potential to produce personal and interpersonal conflict or stress.

Coping with caring is a complex area, but I offers some examples of issues arising from my analysis. Strategies for coping include a sort of strategic conformity which means avoiding trouble, and attempting to deal with guilt caused by the need to 'grumble'. It is particularly important to view the section on caring as a element in the nurses' coping strategy since brilliant care and the covert liking which I documented earlier are examples of how interlinked the coping approaches are with the daily social processes of nursing.

The coping strategies of patients, namely negotiating, struggling and acquiescing are the principal processes through which they cope with their situation. The core elements of the patients' strategies, however, when seen as part of a dialogue between nurses and patients, begin to form a process theory of social judgement and its context. In the final chapter I aim to review the main elements of my account of what I believe to be a substantive theory of the process of social judgement as I discovered it on Howarth Ward. I will endeavour to draw into the discussion the importance of power as both a context and consequence of social judgement, and will conclude with an account of implications of my argument for practice, education, theory and research.

12 Conclusion: a theory of social judgement

In this chapter I intend to restate the essence of my account of the process of social judgement in Howarth Ward. I plan to illustrate the importance that a conception of social judgement has for the understanding of the power relations between social actors in the ward. I will consequently discuss influential views of power as a backcloth against which social judgement must be seen.

The concept of social judgement

Whilst others, such as Roth (1972) have referred to the evaluation of the social worth of others as 'moral evaluation' this term has a different meaning to philosophers, one of the assessment of the morality of an idea or a course of action. Generally therefore, I have found it useful to refer to the labelling of persons as 'good' or 'bad', 'popular' or 'unpopular' as social judgement. This is not to say that there is not a moral component to this activity, since there may be both positive and negative consequences for an individual so labelled. Further, some sociologists utilise the term 'moral career' to refer to the biography of a person in terms of their social worth as judged by others. In choosing the term social judgement for the process which I see as the main focus of this study, I do not wish to add to the semantic confusion. I trust however that my use of the term is clear in its context and by means of the definition I offer.

The elaboration of a notion of the process of social judgement inevitably depends upon some consideration of the social context in which it occurs. I have endeavoured to discuss key elements of the social context, and as my analysis developed the concepts of power and control became of importance. I therefore focus upon these as major aspects of the social context in this study.

Earlier I discuss some of the strategies which are used by nurses and patients in order to derive, consolidate and exercise their power. In this chapter I will draw upon theoretical conceptions of power to help illuminate the place which social judgement may have in an analysis of professional-client power relations.

The process of social judgement

Being labelled as a good patient or a bad one, as popular or unpopular has commonly been seen as a result of traits possessed by patients, such as having a sense of humour, having a particular illness, or failing to adhere to the obligations in the Parsonian conception of the sick role. In common with Kelly and May (1982) who first attacked these reductive explanations from an interactionist perspective, I believe I show both from the evidence I present and from the analysis of a wider interactionist literature, that the traits theory is inadequate. Rather, it may be the case that no predictive theory of labelling people in a social context is possible. Certainly attempts to quantify the variables said to predict unpopularity seem to have failed (see Stockwell, 1972). In consequence, when it became apparent to me in my early fieldwork on Howarth Ward that unpopularity of patients was of major concern to nursing staff, I made this the focus of my analysis and collection of data.

The analysis and collection of my data were guided by the techniques developed by Strauss and others and called grounded theory (Glaser and Strauss, 1967; Strauss and Corbin, 1990). Consequently I will claim that, following their use of the term, my account of the process of labelling people as good or bad, or social judgement, is a substantive theory. That is to say, it is a descriptive and explanatory account of an important social phenomenon in a particular context, Howarth Ward. I make suggestions about possible relationships between factors, or variables, but make no claim that these relationships are necessarily causal.

Because of the profound complexity of the social world, and the necessarily selective nature of my account of the phenomena I describe, this 'theory' represents my interpretation of events, based on the best analysis I could make of the data I obtained. I have attempted to render explicit the theoretical and experiential orientations which guided me so that my 'theory' may be judged accordingly.

A social judgement theory

Social judgement is inextricably linked with the social processes of the management of care. The official version of the management of care is the nursing process, which is a staged process of assessing the need for care, planning, implementing and evaluating nursing activities (Kratz, 1979). My fieldwork as a participant observer in the role of qualified nurse on

Howarth Ward, and interviews with the staff, caused me to modify this substantially. The process of social judgement, which took place alongside the planning and delivery of nursing actions, also incorporated assessing. This form of assessment, however, included the use of stereotypes, and then went on to be a process in which nurses and patients presented themselves as they thought fit so that their future interactions would meet their own and others' expectations. This meant for example that nurses made it clear that they had the right to survey (examine) and control the patients' intimate bodily functions, which immediately clarified the status relations between them. *Assessing* allowed nurses to judge the potential of the patient to contribute to the work of the ward, a type of work rarely rendered explicit or accounted for. Based upon the process of assessment, both nurses and patients form an opinion of each other, which may be modified through *negotiation*.

Patients can re-negotiate their labels, through the performance of *work*, that is, making the work of nurses easier, or by adopting a wide range of tactics such as humour, compliance, or the giving of gifts. Some gifts are symbolic, such as praise. In all negotiations, whether verbal or non-verbal, staff have the most influence and are the most likely to satisfy their goals. Where they do not, they have the sanction of unpopularity to bestow, which can mean avoidance by nurses or explicit conflict.

Struggling, a form of interpersonal conflict between nurses and patients, is far from idealised conceptions of the nursing process. Here in particular the overlap between struggling to modify a known image or self-presentation and struggling to achieve basic goals such as independence is greatest. Generally patients are seriously disempowered in hospital despite the rhetoric of individualised care that accompanies the nursing process (Littlewood, 1991). Nevertheless some strategies are available to patients to achieve their aims through struggling, such as complaining to managers and through appealing to the anxieties that the nurses have, such as not being allowed to give essential pressure area care. As in other areas of social life, struggling is likely to lead to a negative reputation, but then some patients know that they have this anyway, so have little to lose.

Acquiescing is the process of going along with the wishes of others in the context of social judgement. It can be the acceptance of a negative label as unavoidable, one that must be borne. Clearly too, it is related to 'compliance' which is the acceptance of medical and nursing prescriptions. I suggest that the overall process of management of care in a climate of social judgement is calculated to achieve acquiescence with nursing goals. Further I argue that, whatever the recent claims to autonomy of nursing staff, nursing goals are explicitly or implicitly related to the furtherance of medical prescriptions and goals as Freidson (1970) and Turner (1987) have suggested.

The importance of acquiescing is that it illustrates the considerable power that health professionals continue to exercise over their patients and the potential for morally dubious conduct to remain unchallenged. An overview of relevant concepts is presented in the accompanying Table 5 on page 178.

Table 5: Some key concepts in the process of social judgement

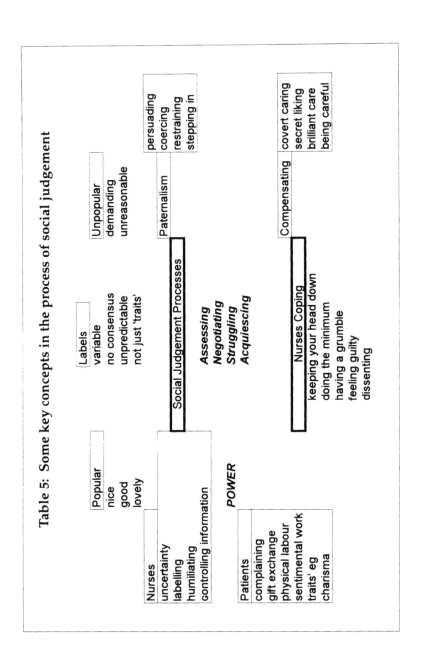

Power and social judgement

As I undertook my analysis it became clearer to me that power is indeed a central concept. I have already drawn briefly upon theories of power which attempt to explain the tactics and strategies people adopt in health care situations. However I feel it appropriate to explore the idea a little more.

In *Power: A Radical View*, Steven Lukes (1974) argues that power is a concept that is "ineradicably value dependent" and is "essentially contested". In a later work (Lukes, 1986), he observes that the search for an all embracing definition of power is a mistake. He suggests that two of the main interests of thinkers and analysts of power are first, the outcomes of power, and second the locus of power. In his (1986) introduction to a collection of papers by some of the foremost writers, he asks questions which extend the discussion of power well beyond the obvious. He summarily dismisses Bertrand Russell's (1938) view of power as "the production of intended effects" with the question: "Is power the actual production of such effects or the capacity to produce them?" He continues his attack with the suggestion that the effects need not be intended for power to be involved, and gives the example of making investment decisions which might put people in or out of work. This example illustrates that even when some luck is involved it may still be appropriate to speak of power. In considering the relations between people in the analysis of power, Lukes asks further searching questions. One of these is "... am I powerful if I can only produce such (intended) effects at enormous cost, say by sacrificing my life...?" (p1).

Lukes (1986) illustrates the lack of concept clarity which pervades the literature, and seems pessimistic that it can be much improved because of the very different perspectives and assumptions brought to bear upon the discussions. Nevertheless it is clear to me how examination of some of these perspectives on power can illuminate and clarify, or at least cause me to think about the clarity or otherwise of my own view of power and related ideas like authority and coercion. For example, when I helped to coerce Sam Read to have an enema I clearly exercised power over him. The justification of this use (or abuse) of power is less certain.

Parsons (1963) sees power as a resource in a social system. It is analogous to money, and he sees it as neither sinister nor beneficent. It is merely a commodity to be used in the achievement of what Parsons sees as the collective goals of the group or social system. Parsons, therefore, tends to see power as inevitably legitimate. This is because, in Parsons' view, it is exercised by people who are the agreed leaders of the society and who necessarily further the goals of the system. Of course this may be through the use of negative sanctions (but people in general will want this). From his functionalist perspective Parsons refuses to see any place in his theory for the illegitimate use of power. Parsons then, would have conceived of the use of professional power of the type present in the instance of the enema with Sam Read, or in the restraint of Robert Munro as legitimate.

Hannah Arendt (1958) discusses power in her comprehensive treatise on *"The Human Condition"*, and in a further work *"On Violence"* (1969). Whilst Lukes (1986) ascribes to Arendt a collective view of power, she could not be described as a functionalist. Lukes means to say that Arendt, like Parsons, sees power as possible only in the context of human relations. Arendt's communications view of power is broadly that it is not important to know who rules whom. Rather, Arendt sees power as something of which:

> ...all political organisations are manifestations and materialisations of power; they petrify and decay as soon as the living power of the people ceases to uphold them. (1969:62)

Arendt (1958) emphasises the notion that power is in some way independent of material factors, either of number or means. By this she means that strength, and force (both of which are measurable) do not necessarily correlate with power. History, she reminds us, is full of small poor countries getting the better of large rich ones. Of course more recent events in Vietnam and Afghanistan lend some support to her hypothesis. Arendt argues that the only indispensable material factor in the generation of power is the living together of people. Even so, power is potentially temporary and is as unreliable as people's opinions. In this respect she departs even further from Parsons (1963), because she is suggesting an essentially socially constructed nature for power. Arendt seems to believe that power is ascribed and exercised through the use of language rather than the use of force. Force, or violence, may be used to the same ends, but they are not in her view power. Indeed she observes that whilst power and force may occur together, they have an essentially opposite nature. By this she means that commonly the use of great force or violence means that power, in her sense of the word, is absent. Here we return to the point of agreement with Parsons (1963), that true power in some way reflects agreement among persons involved as to who may exercise power and in what circumstances.

In the context of health care practice and social judgement, it is possible to see how Arendt's communications concept of power is of value. She argues that power is only truly present when force is not necessary. Therefore from her point of view the use of coercion or physical force to engage the compliance of a patient might indicate a loss of power.

However, in view of her notion of the agreement of those involved, such tactics would be seen as the exercise of medical or nursing power provided that people in general did not challenge these tactics, or indeed encouraged them. This would define the situation as a legitimate exercise of power. In this context Arendt's view of authority is similarly based. She sees authority as deriving from respect, not merely formal status, so that the authority that nurses and others have to achieve their aims is based upon the respect that patients have for health professionals. This respect and the authority it bestows (or the possibility for the exercise of power), is socially constructed. Arendt, then, would broadly support an interactionist conception of power which would have the implication that opinions of social value (social judgement) would play an important part in the social construction of power relations. Arendt's view of power as socially constructed could help to explain how patients whose power to resist nursing and medical interventions was greater than trait theories would predict. An example would be Doug Whitbread who maintained both his popularity and his ability to not comply with treatment despite being in an apparently weak position according to criteria of popularity evident in previous research.

A British theorist of some influence today, and whose work deals extensively with power, is Anthony Giddens. In *Studies in Social and Political Theory* (1977) Giddens attempts to synthesise a general theory of social interaction which avoids the dualism common in sociological accounts. In proposing a theory of structuration he hopes to make redundant ideas of a conflict between epistemologies such as positivism and phenomenology. In relation to power, Giddens has provided a good deal of analysis both of his own and of others' accounts. If it is fair to tie him to one definition of power, it is 'transformative capacity'. He goes on to say that :

All the processes of the structuration (production and reproduction) of systems of social interaction involve three elements: the communication of meaning, the exercise of power, and the evaluation and judgement of conduct. (Giddens, 1977:132)

On this view Giddens clearly supports the idea that the judgement of human conduct, and the language used to communicate the meaning thereof, are clear sources of power in social relations. More recently Giddens (1991) has discussed how symbolic modes of expressing power differentials are "deeply implicated in day-to-day practical activities often of the most mundane kind" (p216). He suggests that ethnography is an integral aspect of social research endeavour to reflect and illuminate such matters. It is therefore clear that Giddens' basic concepts have potential to

181

tie together many of the elements of a theory of social judgement, and he acutely observes the close relation that seems to exist between evaluative labelling and power of some sort.

Whilst he is very aware of the redundancy of the protracted search for a satisfactory definition of power, Steven Lukes (1986) takes an essentially Marxian view which draws upon the critical theory of the Frankfurt School. According to Hoy (1986):

> To Lukes, power is essentially 'power over'. The social scientific question is, then, how to study the exercise of power-over when so defined. (Hoy, 1986:125)

Lukes' (1974) radical model of power goes beyond the largely consensual views of Parsons and Arendt to examine what the exercise of power (over) prevents people from doing and even thinking. Lukes' model is radical in the sense that it makes the assumption that individuals (or groups) have responsibility for the exercise (or not) of their power. Hoy (1986) summarises Lukes' position thus:

> Lukes sides with those who link power to human agency. His reason is that to talk about an exercise of power is necessarily to assume that it is in the exerciser's power to act differently. (Hoy, 1986:126)

Such a view of power has much in common with what Harris (1974) calls "the Marxist conception of violence". That is to say that as much responsibility attaches to a decision not to prevent violence as to use it. Indeed as Harris argues, the idea of acts and omissions doctrine is not at all new. Its application to fundamental concepts like power is, however, in the current context at least, seen as radical.

Lukes' opinion then, is that whatever the difficulties of definition, it would be a mistake to ascribe too deterministic a position to power in the social world. If Lukes can be classified at all, he holds a Marxist view, that the exercise of power can be both beneficent and maleficent, and that responsibility can often be ascribed both for its exercise and its effects. The implication of Lukes' view then, is that social actors should be aware of the impact they may have, for example, in choosing to use a particular form of language to describe someone. This is because we bear responsibility for the consequences of exercising such a choice. In acknowledging that where there is power, there is also struggle, Lukes' conception of power and responsibility for human action has a good deal to offer the analysis of both the nursing and social judgement processes. This is because each of these has previously been described, in theoretical works at least, in idealised and consensual terms (see Orem, 1980).

Whilst acknowledging the influence of Michel Foucault, Lukes departs substantially, as do most writers, from the position Foucault establishes in most of his work. In "Discipline and Punish" (1991, first published 1975), Foucault develops the notion that power and knowledge are related and indeed conceptually inseparable (for his purposes at least). He is also explicit that power is what he terms diffuse, that is it is not held by individuals. Foucault argues that power and its sequelae, subjugation, coercion and discipline are as much given by the subjugated as taken by the powerful. He takes an historical perspective, showing how it is that extreme forms of punishment and restraint are no longer necessary in order to control the members of society. Such tactics live on, however, in more subtle forms of control and surveillance. Foucault argues that the growth of scientific knowledge, framed in positivist terms, has replaced the severest forms of social control applied to the mentally ill, to criminals, and to the poor. He rejects the notion, however, that this is in any way progress. He suggests that the means for the limitation of freedom of individual expression are just as widespread. Indeed he seems to see the relative subtlety of the application of power through professional knowledge as less honest and more sinister.

The power of health professionals is expressed through what he terms the 'clinical gaze', a concept of great importance to Foucault. This notion implies not only the medical (and nursing) profession's power to define reality in its terms, but to examine, diagnose, to observe and even to restrain all those it defines as within its proper sphere of influence. In this example it is possible to see the gaze, and therefore power, as diffuse in the way that Foucault describes. It can be and is exercised by individuals or groups, but transcends them historically. Social judgement, to Foucault, would be an aspect of the gaze, that is a means through which professional power/knowledge is maintained. In this it is tied to other strategies utilised by nurses and such as humiliation and constant observation. Humiliation is nowhere mentioned as the legitimate aim of intimate nursing procedures, but it is without doubt the patient's experience of the control and observation by nurses of bodily elimination of waste.

Hoy (1986) argues that whilst Foucault, like Lukes (1974), is keen to analyse how it is that people exercise power, he is unlike him in his insistence that the exercisers of power do not themselves possess it. Rather, the whole fabric of society is seen as both the source and the outcome of power/knowledge, but over which professionals through their mythologising of science have increasing control.

To summarise then, it is possible to view the clinical context of a hospital ward in terms of power held or exercised by individuals and groups. At the micropolitical level, explanations are to be found in the interactionist sociology of work perspective, the related positions of

Freidson's (1970) 'sociology of applied knowledge' and Littlewood's (1991) notions of the importance of control of basic body functions and the consequent humiliation as a tactic for deriving power. Examples in relation to nurses are their subordination to both medicine and general managers, whilst at the same time maintaining their influence over patients through control of information and of the patient's body.

As in other respects, the Parsonian (1963) functionalist perspective is found seriously wanting since it assumes consensus when the evidence of both research literature and data is to the contrary. Arendt's view that power must evolve out of human relations is very helpful. Her idea is that authority is dependent upon respect, but the question of whose respect is necessary (or perceived as more important) for the health professional such as a nurse or doctor remains. As I believe I show, the respect of the client is commonly seen as less valuable despite the rhetoric offered by the professions.

In some ways Foucault's work is comparable to that of Ivan Illich (1976). It is polemical, and contains illustrative examples which capture the imagination. In particular, Foucault's notion that we are enmeshed in a web of power which professionals gain access to in order to control their clients helps to illuminate the power that nurses and others in health care are able to exercise in order to secure compliance.

I am left having examined some key notions of power with a sense that, as Lukes (1986) argues, the search for a tight definition is fraught with problems. I have attempted to use the word in a context in which its meaning is clear for that part of the text. In some ways, the differing conceptions of power are not in competition. Seen at the most observable point of its exercise, the nurse-patient relationship, the locus and the outcomes of the exercise of power are evident. It is also possible to see how it is useful to conceive of power in the form of a diffuse context which both arises out of and facilitates human relations and aims. Such a perspective would help to illustrate how it is that nurses putting patients in the bath is, whether they realise it or not, the exercise of power on behalf of, say, the medical profession or indeed something which might be called society.

Having reviewed conceptions of power as they seem to apply to my argument, I would be unhappy with any view which did not incorporate a sense of struggle, since I argue that this element of the process of social judgement (and of nursing) is the most neglected. Even in the work of Strauss and his colleagues (such as Strauss et al, 1982a) which I otherwise find so useful, the concept of conflict as a key element in their social theory is less pronounced than it might be.

The consequences of social judgement

I believe I make clear that evaluative labels are not permanent, and may vary between individuals. By this I mean that there may be an official version and an unofficial one so that a patient apparently unpopular in the ward report given by the nurse in charge may not be seen as such by other nurses, especially the students. As a consequence of this, nurses attempt to compensate for the official negative label by giving particularly good care, or by paying special attention to certain patients. Sometimes this activity has to be covert, since students cannot normally afford to challenge the orthodoxy of the official label too openly. Coping with this dissonance between official and unofficial versions of reality is, however, something students learn very quickly since this applies also to the way nursing care and procedures are taught and then experienced in the reality of the ward (Melia, 1987). In order to cope, nurses 'keep their head down' and 'have a grumble' to each other. Sometimes, however, nurses will be able to dissent up to a point provided that their reputation is already safe, through hard work and attention to detail, for example.

Another consequence of social judgement, if sometimes an indirect one, is paternalistic restraint and coercion to acquiesce to nursing procedures which are defined by the nurses as important.

The moral climate of Howarth ward, then, incorporated the evaluation of the social worth of individuals and the exercise of power in both beneficent and paternalistic ways. If autonomy is an important principle of human relations in general and health care in particular (Chadwick and Russell, 1989), then some nursing practices override this principle. To say that such action is harmful at this point would go beyond my data. The question of the claimed beneficence of paternalistic care is, however, an important one and worthy of substantial investigation from both empirical and philosophical points of view.

Having summarised the main elements of my account of the process of social judgement and some of the factors which relate to it, I now intend to discuss some of the specific implications of this work for practice, education, theory and research.

Implications for nursing practice, education, theory and research

In discussing implications it is inevitable that I go beyond my data to speculate as if the issues arising in this study are more generally applicable than it is justifiable to claim. I do however write as an experienced nurse and teacher with, I hope, an amount of sensitivity to how nursing is practised in the wider context. An ethnography of one ward is clearly vulnerable to the criticism that its discoveries are not applicable to other settings. This book is an attempt to provide detailed insights into the phenomenon of social judgement with which many nurses will identify.

Nursing practice

The main implication for practice which Stockwell (1984) identifies based upon her study published in 1972 is:

> that by being kind, attentive and nice to people when they are being "nasty" you are much more likely to improve their behaviour than by being curt, cross and ignoring them. (p1)

This is all very well, and is a principle that most nurses would have been taught in introductory or foundation courses. 'The customer is always right' ideology is laudable in itself, but most of us cannot keep it up. It is something we would all probably like to do, but it doesn't work out in practice. Indeed a good deal of the guilt that nurses seem to feel if they do award people negative labels may arise out of the dissonance they feel knowing that they should have higher standards. Whilst Stockwell's (1984) recommendation has some merit in individual circumstances, as Bradby (1990) shows, I intend to offer some other possible ways forward in managing care in a context of virtually inevitable social judgement.

Ward (change of shift) reports

The standard format for care planning and communication between nurses about patients continues to be the office-based ward report. In my study a good deal of the judgemental discussion of patients took place in this forum, and the resulting labels therefore had a sort of official nature from which less experienced nurses had difficulty dissenting.

Bedside rather than office-based reports are not new. They have been common practice in intensive care units and I experienced them in the early 1970's in a neurosurgical unit. Their prevalence in such units probably indicated that it was assumed that patients could not hear or did not care what was said about them. Both assumptions were of course fallacious. Placing the main forum for communication about patients by their bedside where they can hear what is said about them ought to cause nursing and other staff to be less judgemental in their communications. Patients and perhaps relatives would have the opportunity to challenge the prevailing view even if, as powerless as many patients are, they chose not to exercise this right. Two key questions remain. If patients are present at the ward report, how will nurses and others keep the diagnosis and/or prognosis secret from them? This begs the question: should they?

Care plans

Related to this and possibly more controversial is the practice of allowing patients access to their care plans. Again the notion is not new and this happens in some areas, but the practice is not widespread and probably the less so the more acute the illness is deemed to be. Allowing clients to be fully involved in their care and the decisions relating to it must have this as a first and important step.

It seems to me that nothing would prevent the 'silent conspiracy' described by Field (1989) should it be really in the client's interest for secrets to be kept. However the need to arrange a covert discussion of such matters outside normal business or to keep vital information out of the plan of care might at least change the emphasis from one in which almost all communication between professionals is closed to one in which most is open.

Recognising the emotional labour of care

Nicky James (1989) and Pam Smith (1992) have drawn special attention to the relatively unrecognised emotional work involved in care. The aim of so much of the rhetoric of the nursing process, and newer methods of organising care such as team nursing and primary nursing, is ostensibly to humanise nurse-patient relationships by breaking down traditional barriers such as a professional distance and task allocation. In identifying task orientation, hierarchical relationships and large social distance between patients and nurses, the early work by Menzies (1960) was drawing attention to the fact that these mechanisms act as defences against the anxieties which are a consequence of unsupported and protracted emotional labour. The so-called 'new nursing' effectively removes some or all of these defences without necessarily proposing an alternative way of coping.

In Howarth Ward a good deal of effort had gone into the provision of individualised care on a team basis, and nurses could already see that working closely with the same patients over a long period of time was more stressful than just having tasks to complete. If commenting on the patients' supposed characters played a part in dealing with this greater closeness it is hardly surprising. The implications of this are that the managerial imperative to implement primary nursing with all speed to meet performance review objectives could cause further breakdown in the defences that those directly giving the care have available to them.

It is important therefore that greater thought be given to the strategies which might be adopted in better preparing nursing staff for emotional labour and in supporting them when they are doing it. I believe that even since the greater emphasis on communication skills training in nursing

187

courses, our provision in this field is very basic and requires a good deal of further development, especially as regards self awareness. In particular, there may be benefit in adopting more supportive approaches to mentorship. Currently the main source of emotional support to nursing staff is informal, at home or in the coffee bar. However valuable, this is not coherent or structured. The concept of supervision, in its therapeutic (rather than managerial) sense may be an area of fruitful exploration for general nurses (Butterworth and Faugier, 1992). This model of support allows those engaged in emotional labour to reflect upon their experiences guided by a suitably prepared and objective colleague. Use of the model presupposes an infrastructure and expertise which is not even fully available in mental health units. However, the recognition that much of nursing, however physical it may appear, is really the management of emotions, both one's own and other peoples', may help to press for such resources to be developed.

Apart from some work by Strauss et al (1982a) the implications of the clients' contribution to the emotional division of labour are so far ill-recognised, and it is in this context that some patients are labelled as unpopular. Where self care and independence are clearly ideologies which nurses have taken up, more work remains to be done to establish the clients' perspective more clearly than has been achieved so far (see Waterworth and Luker, 1990).

"Brilliant care"

In an influential work the American Patricia Benner (1984) describes her research into excellent practice. She outlines a model of the development of expertise which depends heavily upon opportunity to reflect upon practice and through which nurses proceed 'from novice to expert'. During my fieldwork period I observed many examples of excellent practice performed by nurses at all levels of development, from first year student to the ward sister. In particular, excellent practice depended upon refined social skills which nurses often possessed as people rather than because they had been taught them in a communication skills workshop. However, these skills and the altruistic ideals to utilise them, surfaced only when it was contextually acceptable to do so. That is, nurses felt their use of special skills or demonstrations of particularly caring behaviours were dependent upon the climate they found themselves in. Otherwise they had to be more covert. This goes for advocacy too. I suggest that most of the time nurses knew when the standard of care provided in any respect was less than they would like, even when it was their own. Creating the environment or the climate in which a reasoned challenge can be made to either a dominant and unfair view of a client or a specific plan of care, will present a major challenge to practitioners in health care. The hope of course is that a superior academic training of the type Project 2000 courses are meant to provide, will solve this problem. However a good deal needs to be done to develop both the medical profession's view of nursing and that of the potential patients, so that clients may increasingly see that there are a number of alternative ways of approaching problems, not merely the one with which patients are usually presented.

Education

My recent background as a lecturer leads me to be cautious about the claims of education to affect practice directly. First I intend to discuss some curriculum issues. The teaching of interpersonal skills has gained in impetus in the last decade (Kagan, 1985). It is important to recognise that in the time available, many such courses provide only an opportunity for group cohesion and basic appreciation of strategies underlying successful interpersonal relations. The opportunity for in-depth exploration of emotions provoked by caring is in this context difficult to provide. Nevertheless, the emotional labour of care, once fully recognised, ought to drive educators and managers of educational resources to identify both expertise and curriculum time to explore such matters. Unfortunately the emotional cost of care is most easily counted as absenteeism and attrition rates. Solutions proposed for the former are usually coercive, such as having to provide medical evidence and to report to a senior manager. The latter has commonly been seen as unavoidable (Buchan, 1992).

In common with communication skills, courses in assertiveness and stress management have been suggested by various sources (Davidson, 1985). There is no doubt that nurses are insufficiently assertive and experience substantial stress in achieving their goals of care in the context of emotional labour. However, new forms of education and training which focus upon the improvement of the skills or expertise of the nurse inevitably individualise responsibility for the situation. They presume that the experiencing of nursing as stressful is merely a skill deficit in the nurse. It would be wrong therefore to expect too much of these methods without attention to wider socio-political issues such as resource management, skill mixes, and interprofessional relationships, notably with the medical profession and the new post-Griffiths professional managers.

The broad implication of my argument is that education, especially of clinical and managerial levels of staff should be multi-disciplinary for nurses and doctors. In this way some wider appreciation of the emotional labour of nursing, a form rarely experienced by other occupations, might be gained.

A further specific development for which my study provides support, is that health professionals and nurses in particular need to have a greater

189

opportunity to debate and to examine a wider spectrum of moral positions and perspectives than currently. A good deal of concern was expressed by my respondents about such matters as coercion, restraint, and excessive treatment. These and other issues are important from day to day, and my limited evidence is that respect for the autonomy of persons is not so prevalent as might be believed. Strategies as diverse as humiliation and physical restraint work in concert with judgemental labelling to render patients relatively powerless to influence their situation. This can be over small matters such as whether to submit to a bath, or very great ones such as deciding to comply with painful and uncomfortable procedures. I am therefore arguing for a greater emphasis in curricula on exploring the moral philosophy of health care and particularly of a type which encourages debate both of the rationale for actions and of the emotions they provoke in those who provide the care.

There is a current climate of maximum managerial efficiency in use of resources, centralisation and amalgamation of educational provision, reduction in intakes of student nurses and consequently of teachers. I am therefore not confident that such qualitative improvements in educational provision will be easy to justify. On the other hand the emphasis on "quality" in contracts both for service and for education could be a lever for such developments if managed effectively.

My final point about educational implications would be to argue that we have made insufficient progress in what Kramer (1974) termed anticipatory socialisation. By this she meant that much of the stress and the shock of working in the real world can be ameliorated by a certain honesty with students about the clinical reality, and a greater exposure to the now considerable literature of occupational socialisation. This ought to be easier to do with health care sociology having a higher profile in diploma and undergraduate degree programmes. On the other hand, diploma and degree programmes provide less clinical experience to students who may increasingly be seen as well-read but less well prepared for what Kramer (1974) termed 'reality shock' on their transition to the busy and demanding role of staff nurse in a large bureaucracy. Kramer argued for preparation in relevant coping strategies such as seeking peer support and which she began to include in her courses.

Implications for theory and research

In nursing, the word theory has come to represent the idealised notions of nursing practice that have been proposed by nursing theorists such as Orem (1980) and Henderson (1966). Little or none of this type of theory can be said to be grounded in systematic empirical investigation. Rather, many such theories are clearly derived deductively from the biological and behavioural sciences. The strength of deductive generalisations is that the models derived from such theories seem clear, precise, and can easily be described by flow charts. They are theories and models of how things ought to be.

Grounded theory, however, attempts to describe and explain the social world as it is experienced by both the observer and so far as is possible, the other people present. Such theory always requires further development, but it can be rich and illuminating for those with an interest in understanding how things are rather than how things ought to be.

Having offered something of a refutation of the traits theory of social judgement, I also discuss a number of other explanations which have been offered. In the late 1970s and early 1980s some attention was given by British sociologists such as Jeffrey (1979) and Dingwall and Murray (1983) to a reformulation of a sociology of deviance perspective which draws heavily upon Parsonian conception of the sick role. The suggestion was that when patients failed to follow the rules therein, they risked unpopularity. Much of this work was devoted to analysing exceptions, however, and adds weight to the notion that labelling is very complex and contextually determined. English and Morse (1988) seem confined at one level by the traits theory in their conclusions about the nurses' views. When they interviewed clients, however, they derived valuable insights into a more processual explanation of the construction of unpopularity. The process was seen much more in terms of the power relations between nurses and patients and in the context of struggle or conflict rather than consensus. The conceptual framework arising out of my analysis of fieldwork and interviews has a specific focus on labelling or judgement of the worth of persons as a social process. Whilst my theory might be described as early or substantive I believe it offers evidence for a reappraisal of the role of social judgement in the determination of the care given to people in a hospital ward and the decisions made about them.

I am confident of the place of inductive approaches in the generation of knowledge about the social world of nursing and health care. I also benefited somewhat from the structural and procedural guidance offered by Strauss and Corbin (1990) on grounded theory. I suspect that with experience researchers will use these highly structured procedures with greater flexibility and creativity as Glaser and Strauss, when on better terms, originally intended. It will be important not to reduce the importance of intuitive insight in the analysis and interpretation of qualitative data however rigorously concepts are derived and refined from their origins in fieldnotes or transcripts.

I suggest in my discussion of method that nurse researchers have been reluctant to utilise true participant methods. I would now argue further that greater energy should be devoted to research which is participatory in the sense of involving respondents in the research process at all levels. Three arguments support this view. First there is a clear need to raise awareness of research among practitioners and to demystify its purpose and methods. Second, participatory methods can often be seen to offer something directly to respondents and facilitate dialogue between researchers and practitioners and third, participant methods allow the intervention of the health researcher to act to avoid harms and to do good where it would be wrong not to.

This thesis represents only one particular focus, upon social judgement, of the wealth of data which I collected during my study. Examples of questions which arise immediately from this study include:

1.   To what extent is the (relatively unrecognised) physical and sentimental work which patients do essential to the delivery and receipt of care?
2.   In what ways do changes in the explicit ideology of health care, such as self care, affect the process of negotiation of social reputation?
3.   Through what social processes do nurses and others come to behave paternalistically toward their patients?
4.   What would be the consequences of a climate in which explicit judgemental labelling is reduced or discouraged?
5.   What are the consequences of 'new' methods of organising nursing care for the process of social judgement?

Summary

In this Chapter I have drawn together a broad restatement of my account of the process of social judgement as it emerged throughout my analysis of fieldwork in a medical ward at a large general hospital. I have attempted to identify key theoretical issues, notably the relationship which seems to exist between notions of judgemental labelling and the maintenance of a power imbalance between patients and nurses. I argue that social judgement is an aspect of a wider social process by which patients are rendered acquiescent to medical and nursing goals, sometimes in contravention of their own stated wishes.

I have suggested some implications for practice, which include scrutiny of new methods of organising nursing care such as team and primary nursing since these have the possibility of increasing rather than lessening the emotional labour of caring, and more open methods of nurse to nurse reporting. I have also cautiously urged that greater attention could be placed upon interpersonal skills, self awareness and assertiveness training. It is important to recognise, however, that such strategies individualise responsibility for problems which are often situated in wider institutional constraints such as hierarchical power relations between occupations and patients. I am concerned that organisational cost efficiencies resulting from deteriorating teacher:student ratios and amalgamation of Colleges of Nursing into Higher Education may further erode the personal support mechanisms available to students of nursing. However, a more research based and scholarly ethos may also have advantages. With appropriate resources given to student support and an enhanced social and ethical component to the curricula which nurses follow in the Diploma in Higher Education (Project 2000) model and the various Degree programmes, nurses will become more aware of the positive and more patient-centred contribution they can make to the negotiation of arrangements for patient care.

Bibliography

Aamodt, A.M. (1991), 'Ethnography and epistemology: generating nursing knowledge' in Morse, J.M. (Ed.), *Qualitative nursing research: a contemporary dialogue*, Sage, Newbury Park

Abrams, N. (1978), 'A contrary view of the nurse as patient advocate', *Nursing Forum*, XVII, 3, 258-267.

Aggleton, P. and Chalmers, H. (1986), *Nursing models and the nursing process*, MacMillan, London.

Altschul, A.T. (1972), *Patient nurse interaction: a study of interaction patterns in acute psychiatric wards*, Churchill Livingstone, Edinburgh.

Anderson, J.M. (1991), 'The phenomenological perspective', in, Morse, J.M. (ed.) *Qualitative nursing research: a contemporary dialogue*, Sage, Newbury Park.

Arendt, H. (1958), *The human condition*, University of Chicago Press, Chicago.

Arendt, H. (1969), 'Communicative power', in, Lukes, S. (ed.) *Power*, Blackwell, Oxford.

Argyle, M. (1967), *The psychology of interpersonal behaviour*, Penguin, Harmondsworth.

Armitage, S. (1980), 'Non-compliant recipients of health care', *Nursing Times*, 76, 1-3.

Ashworth, P. (1980), *Care to communicate*, Royal College of Nursing, London.

Bailey, M.P. (1985), 'A qualitative research method to study two residences', in, Leininger, M.M. (ed.) *Qualitative research methods in nursing*, Grune and Stratton, Orlando.

Baker, D.E. (1978), *Attitudes of nurses to the care of the elderly*, Unpublished Ph.D Thesis, University of Manchester.

Beardshaw, V. (1981), *Conscientious objectors at work*, Social Audit, London.

Becker, H. (1958), 'Problems of inference and proof in participant observation', *American Sociological Review*, 23, 652-660.

194

Becker, H., Geer, B., Hughes, E.C. and Strauss, A. (1961) *Boys in white: student culture in medical school*, University of Chicago Press, Chicago.

Becker, H.S. and Geer, B. (1969), 'Participant observation and interviewing: a comparison', in, McCall, G.J. and Simmons, J. (eds.) *Issues in participant observation*, Addison Wesley, Reading Mass.

Bell, C. and Encel, S. (eds, 1978), *Inside the whale: ten personal accounts of social research*, Pergamon, Oxford.

Bendall, E. (1975), *So you passed nurse*, Royal College of Nursing, London.

Benjamin, M and Curtis, J. (1981) *Ethics in nursing*, Oxford University Press, New York.

Benner, P. (1984), *From novice to expert: excellence and power in clinical nursing practice*, Addison Wesley, Menlo Park, California.

Benyon, J. (1987), 'Zombies in dressing gowns', in, McKeganey, N.P. and Cunningham-Burley, S. (eds.) *Enter the sociologist: reflections on the practice of sociology*, Avebury, Aldershot.

Birch, J. (1975), *To nurse or not to nurse?*, Royal College of Nursing, London.

Blegen, M.A. and Lawler, E.J. (1989), 'Power and bargaining in authority-client relations', *Research in Political Sociology*, 4, 167-186.

Bogdan, R. and Taylor, S.J. (1975), *Introduction to qualitative research methods: a phenomenological approach to the social sciences*, John Wiley, New York.

Boore, J.R.P. (1978), *Prescription for recovery*, Royal College of Nursing, London.

Bradby, M.B. (1990), 'Status passage into nursing: undertaking nursing care', *Journal of Advanced Nursing*, 15, 1363-1369.

Brand, F.N. and Smith, R.T. (1974), 'Medical care and compliance among the elderly after hospitalisation', *International Journal of Ageing and Human Development*, 5, 4, 331-346.

Brown, G.W. (1973), 'Some thoughts on grounded theory', *The Journal of the British Sociological Association*, 7, 1-16.

Bruyn, S.T. (1966), *The human perspective in sociology: the methodology of participant observation*, Prentice Hall, Englewood Cliffs, New Jersey.

Buchan, J. (1992), 'Nurse manpower planning: role, rationale and relevance', in, Robinson, J., Gray, A. and Elkan, R. (eds.) *Policy issues in nursing*, Open University Press, Milton Keynes.

Buckenham, J.E. and McGrath, G. (1983), *The social reality of nursing*, The Health Science Press, Sydney.

Bulmer, M. (1982), *Social research ethics*, MacMillan, London.

Burgess, R.G. (1982), 'Some role problem in field research', in, Burgess, R.G. (ed.) *Field research: a source book and field manual*, Allen and Unwin, London.

Butterworth, C.A. and Faugier, J. (1992), *Clinical supervision and mentorship in nursing*, Chapman and Hall, London.

Candy, C.E. (1991), 'Not for resuscitation: the student nurses' viewpoint', *Journal of Advanced Nursing*, 16, 138-146.

Cartwright, A. and O'Brien, M. (1976), 'Social class variations in health care and in the nature of general practice consultations', in, Tuckett, D. and Kaufert, J.M. (eds, 1978) *Basic readings in medical sociology*, Tavistock, London.

Cash, K. (1992), *Formal models of nursing, tacit knowledge and expertise in psychiatric nursing*, Unpublished PhD Thesis, University of Manchester.

Chadwick, R. and Russell, J. (1989), 'Hospital discharge of frail elderly people: social and ethical considerations in the discharge decision-making process', *Ageing and Society*, 9, 3, 277-295.

Chalmers, K.I. (1990), *Preventative work with families in the community: a qualitative study of health visiting practice*, Unpublished Ph.D. Thesis, University of Manchester.

Cicourel, A.V. (1964), *Method and measurement in sociology*, Free Press, New York.

Clark, L. (1996a), 'Covert participant observation in a secure unit', *Nursing Times*, 92, 48, 37-40.

Clark, L. (1996b), 'Participant observation in a secure unit: Care, conflict and control', *Nursing Times Research*, 1, 6, 431-441.

Colledge, M.M. (1979), 'Observing nursing: exploration of the familiar', in, Colledge, M.M. and Jones, D. (eds.) *Readings in nursing*, Churchill Livingstone, Edinburgh.

Conrad, P. (1979), 'Types of medical social control', *Sociology of Health and Illness*, 1, 1, 1-11.

Corbin, J.M. and Strauss, A.L. (1985), 'Issues concerning regimen management in the home', *Ageing and Society*, 5, 249-265.

Cormack, D. F. S. (1976), *Psychiatric nursing observed*, Royal College of Nursing, London.

Corner, J. (1991), 'In search of more complete answers to research questions; quantitative versus qualitative methods, is there a way forward?', *Journal of Advanced Nursing*, 16, 718-727.

Crotty, M. (1996), *Phenomenology and nursing research*, Churchill Livingstone, Melbourne.

Davidson, C. (1985), 'The theoretical antecedents to interpersonal skills training', in, Kagan, C. (ed.) *Interpersonal skills in nursing: research and applications*, Croom Helm, London.

Delamont, S. (1987), 'Clean baths and dirty women: pollution beliefs on a gynaecology ward', in, McKeganey, N.P. and Cunningham-Burley, S. (eds.) *Enter the sociologist: reflections on the practice of sociology*, Avebury, Aldershot.

Denzin, N.K. (1970), *The research act: a theoretical introduction to sociological methods*, Aldine, Chicago.

Denzin, N.K. (1992), *Symbolic interactionism and cultural studies*, Blackwell, Oxford.

Department of Health (1989), *Working for patients*, HMSO, London.

Dingwall, R. (1977), *The social organisation of health visitor training*, Unpublished Ph.D. Thesis, University of Aberdeen.

Dingwall, R. (1980), 'Ethics and ethnography', *Sociological Review*, 28, 871-981.

Dingwall, R. and Murray, T. (1983), 'Categorisation in accident departments: 'good' patients, 'bad' patients and 'children' ', *Sociology of Health and Illness*, 5, 2, 127-147.

English, J. and Morse, J.M. (1988), 'The 'difficult' elderly patient: adjustment or maladjustment?', *International Journal of Nursing Studies*, 25, 1, 23-39.

Eysenck, H.J. and Kamin, L. (1981), *Intelligence: the battle for the mind*, MacMillan, London.

Faugier, J. (1981), *The experience of nursing in a specialised unit for the treatment of alcoholic patients*, Unpublished M.Sc. Thesis, University of Manchester.

Faulkner, A. (1979), 'Monitoring nurse-patient communication in a ward', *Nursing Times*, 75, 35, Occasional Papers, 95-96.

Festinger, L. (1957), *A theory of cognitive dissonance*, Harper, New York.

Field, D. (1989), *Nursing the dying*, Routledge, Tavistock.

Field, P. and Morse, J.M. (1985), *Nursing research: qualitative methods*, Croom Helm, London.

Field, P.A. (1990), 'Doing fieldwork in your own culture', in, Morse, J.M. (ed.) *Qualitative nursing research: a contemporary dialogue*, Sage, Newbury Park

Fielding, P. (1986), *Attitudes revisited: an examination of student nurses' attitudes towards old people in hospital*, Royal College of Nursing, London.

Fineman, N. (1991), 'The social construction of non-compliance: a study of health care and social service providers in everyday practice', *Sociology of Health and Illness*, 13, 3, 354-374.

Foucault, M. (1991, first pub. 1975), *Discipline and punish*, Penguin, Harmondsworth.

Fox, D.J. (1982), *Fundamentals of research in nursing*, Appleton Century Crofts, New York.

197

Freidson, E. (1962), 'Dilemmas in the doctor-patient relationship', in, Rose, A.M. (ed.) *Human behaviour and social processes: an interactionist approach*, Routledge and Kegan Paul, London.

Freidson, E. (1970), *Profession of medicine: a study in the sociology of applied knowledge*, Dodd Mead, New York.

Gans, H.J. (1968), 'The participant observer as a human being: observations on the personal aspects of fieldwork', in, Burgess, R.G. (ed, 1982) *In the field: an introduction to field research*, Allen and Unwin, London.

Gasek, G. (1980), 'How to handle the crotchety, elderly patient', *Nursing (USA)*, 80, 47-48.

Geddie, W. (ed, 1964), *Chambers' Twentieth Century Dictionary*, Chambers, Edinburgh.

Geer, B. (1969), 'First days in the field: a chronicle of research in progress', in, McCall, G. and Simmons, J. (eds.) *Issues in participant observation*, Addison Wesley, Reading, Mass.

Gibb, H. and O'Brien, B. (1990), 'Jokes and reassurance are not enough: ways in which nurses relate through conversation with elderly clients', *Journal of Advanced Nursing*, 15, 1389-1401.

Giddens, A. (1968), ' 'Power' in the recent writings of Talcott Parsons', *Sociology*, 2, 257-270.

Giddens, A. (1977), *Studies in social and political theory*, Hutchinson, London.

Giddens, A. (1991), 'Structuration theory: past, present and future', in, Bryant, C.G.A. and Jary, D. (eds.) *Giddens' theory of structuration: a critical appreciation*, Routledge, London.

Glaser, B.G. and Strauss, A.L. (1964), 'The social loss of dying patients', *American Journal of Nursing*, 64, 6, 119-120.

Glaser, B.G. and Strauss, A.L. (1967), *The discovery of grounded theory*, Aldine, Chicago.

Glaser, B. (1992), *Basics of grounded theory analysis*, Sociology Press, Mill Valley, California.

Goffman, E. (1959), *The presentation of self in everyday life*, Penguin, Harmondsworth.

Goffman, E. (1963), *Stigma: notes on the management of spoiled identity*, Prentice Hall, New York.

Goffman, E. (1968), *Asylums*, Penguin, Harmondsworth.

Goffman, E. (1971), *The presentation of self in everyday life*, Penguin, Harmondsworth.

Gold, R. (1958), 'Roles in sociological field observations', *Social Forces*, 36, 3, 217-223.

Greenwood, J. (1984), 'Nursing research: a position paper', *Journal of Advanced Nursing*, 9, 1, 77-82.

Griffin, A.P. (1980), 'Philosophy and nursing', *Journal of Advanced Nursing*, 5, 3, 261-272.

Habenstein, R.A. and Christ, E.A. (1963), *Professionalizer, Traditionalizer and Utilizer*, University of Missouri, Columbia.

Habermas, J. (1977), 'Hannah Arendt's communications concept of power', in, Lukes, S. (ed. 1986) *Power*, Blackwell, Oxford.

Hammersley, M. and Atkinson, P. (1983), *Ethnography: principles in practice*, Routledge, London.

Hammersley, M. (1990), *Reading ethnographic research: a critical guide*, Longman, London.

Hammersley, M. (1992), *What's wrong with ethnography?* Routledge, London.

Harris, J. (1974), 'The Marxist conception of violence', *Philosophy and Public Affairs*, 3, 2, 192-220.

Harris, J. (1985), *The value of life: an introduction to medical ethics*, Routledge, London.

Hart, L. (1991), 'A ward of my own: social organisation and identity among hospital domestics', in, Holden P. and Littlewood, J. (eds.) *Anthropology and nursing*, Routledge, London.

Hawthorne, P. (1974), *Nurse, I want my mummy!*, Royal College of Nursing, London.

Henderson, V. (1966), *The nature of nursing*, MacMillan, New York.

Hewison, A. (1995), 'Power of language in a ward for the care of older people', *Nursing Times*, 91, 21, 32-33.

Hochschild, A.R. (1983), *The managed heart: commercialization of human feeling*, University of California Press, Berkeley.

Hoy, D.C. (1986), 'Power, repression, progress: Foucault, Lukes and the Frankfurt School', in, Hoy, D.C. (ed.) *Foucault: a critical reader*, Blackwell, Oxford.

Hughes, E. (1958), *Twenty thousand nurse tell their story*, Lippincott, Philadelphia.

Illich, I. (1976), *Limits to medicine*, Marion Boyars, London.

Ingham, R. and Fielding, P. (1985), 'A review of the nursing literature on attitudes towards old people', *International Journal of Nursing Studies*, 22, 3, 171-181.

James, N. (1989), 'Emotional labour: skill and work in the social regulation of feelings', *The Sociological Review*, 37, 1, 15-42.

James, V. (1986), *Care and work in nursing the dying: a participant study in a continuing care unit*, Unpublished Ph.D. Thesis, University of Aberdeen.

Jeffrey, R. (1979), 'Normal rubbish: deviant patients in casualty departments', *Sociology of Health and Illness*, 1, 1, 90-107.

Johnson, B.E.D. (1987), *The interruption as moral evaluation: an analysis of nursing interactions regarding levels of client care in the midst of conflicting pressures for change*, Unpublished Ph.D. Dissertation, University of Minnesota, Microfilm 8713076.

Johnson, J.M. (1975), *Doing field research*, Collier MacMillan, London.

Johnson, M.L. (1975), 'Old age and the gift relationship', *New Society*, 13th March.

Johnson, M. (1983), *Nurses' values and nurse training: a pilot survey of the values of student nurses*, Unpublished M.Sc. Thesis, University of Manchester.

Johnson, M. (1990), 'Natural sociology and moral questions in nursing: can there be a relationship?', *Journal of Advanced Nursing*, 15, 12, 1358-1362.

Johnson, M. (1992), 'A silent conspiracy: ethical issues of participant observation in nursing research', *International Journal of Nursing Studies*, 29, 2, 213-223.

Johnson, M. (1996), 'Student nurses: novices or practitioners of 'brilliant care'?', *Nursing Times*, June 26th, 92, 24, 34-37.

Johnson, M. (1997), 'Observations on the neglected concept of intervention in nursing research', *Journal of Advanced Nursing*, 25, 1, 23-29.

Johnson, T. J. (1972), *Professions and power*, MacMillan, London.

Jones, J.A. (1985), 'A study of nurse tutors' conceptualisations of their ward teaching role', *Journal of Advanced Nursing*, 10, 4, 349-360.

Kagan, (ed, 1985), *Interpersonal skills in nursing: research and applications*, Croom Helm, London,

Kappeli, S. (1984), *Towards a practice theory of the relationship of self care needs, nursing needs and nursing care in the hospitalised elderly*, Unpublished Ph.D. Thesis, University of Manchester.

Kelly, M.P. and May, D. (1982), 'Good and bad patients: a review of the literature and a theoretical critique', *Journal of Advanced Nursing*, 7, 147-156.

Kershaw, B. and Salvage, J. (1986), *Models for nursing*, Wiley, London.

Ketefian, S. (1988), *'Moral reasoning and ethical practice in nursing: an integrative review'*, National League for Nursing, New York.

Knowles, M. (1978), *The adult learner: a neglected species*, 2nd edition, Gulf, Houston.

Kohlberg, L. (1969), 'A cognitive developmental approach to socialisation', in, Goslin, D. (ed.) *Handbook of socialisation*, Rand McNally, Chicago.

Kohnke, M.F. (1982), 'Advocacy: what is it?', *Nursing and Health Care*, 3, 6, 314-318.

Kramer, M. (1974), *Reality shock: why nurses leave nursing*, Mosby, St. Louis.

Kratz, C.R. (1974), *Problems of the long term sick in the community*, Unpublished Ph.D. Thesis, University of Manchester.

Kratz, C.R. (ed, 1979), *The nursing process*, Bailliere Tindall, London.

Kuhn, M.H. (1962), 'The interview and the professional relationship', in, Rose, A.M. (ed.) *Human behaviour and social processes: an interactional approach*, Routledge and Kegan Paul, London.

Layder, D. (1993), *New strategies in social research*, Polity Press, Cambridge.

Leininger, M.M. (1970), *Nursing and Anthropology: two worlds blend*, John Wiley, Cambridge.

Leininger, M.M. (1985), 'Nature, rationale and importance of qualitative research methods in nursing', in, Leininger, M.M. (ed.) *Qualitative research methods in nursing*, Grune and Stratton, Orlando.

Lelean, S. (1973), *Ready for report, nurse?*, Royal College of Nursing, London.

Lemert, E.M. (1967), 'Deviance and social control', in, Worsley, P. (ed,1978), *Modern sociology*, 2nd. edition, Penguin, Harmondsworth.

Littlewood, J. (1991), 'Care and ambiguity: towards a concept of nursing', in, Holden, P. and Littlewood, J. (eds.) *Anthropology and nursing*, Routledge, London.

Lofland, J. (1971), *Analysing social settings*, Wadsworth, California.

Lorber, J. (1975), 'Good patients and problem patients: conformity and deviance in a general hospital', *Journal of Health and Social Behavior*, 16, 213-225.

Luker, K.A. (1984), 'Reading nursing: the burden of being different', *International Journal of Nursing Studies*, 21, 1, 1-7.

Lukes, S. (1974), *Power: a radical view*, MacMillan, London.

Lukes, S. (ed, 1986), *Power*, Blackwell, Oxford.

Lynch-Sauer, J. (1985), 'Using a phenomenological research method to study nursing phenomena', in, Leininger, M.M. (ed.) *Qualitative research methods in nursing*, Grune and Stratton, Orlando.

McCall, G.J. and Simmons, J. (eds, 1969), *Issues in participant observation*, Addison Wesley, Reading, Mass.

McFarlane, J.K. (1971), *The proper study of the nurse*, Royal College of Nursing, London.

McFarlane, J.K. and Castledine, G. (1982), *A guide to the practice of nursing using the nursing process*, Mosby, London.

McIntosh, J. (1977), *Communication and awareness in a cancer ward*, Croom Helm, London.

McKeganey, N. (1984), ' "No doubt she's really a little princess": a case study of trouble in a therapeutic community', *Sociological Review*, 328-348.

Mauss, M. (1954), 'The gift, Free Press', quoted in, Johnson, M.L. (1979) 'Old age and the gift relationship', *New Society*, 13th March.

May, C. (1992), 'Nursing work, nurses' knowledge, and the subjectification of the patient', *Sociology of Health and Illness*, 14, 4, 472-487.

May, D. and Kelly, M.P. (1982), 'Chancers, pests and poor wee souls: the problem of legitimation in psychiatric nursing', *Sociology of Health and Illness*, 4, 3, 280-301.

Meighan, R. (Ed,1986), *A sociology of educating*, Holt Rinehart and Winston, London.

Melia, K.M. (1981), *Student nurses' accounts of their work and training: a qualitative analysis*, Unpublished Ph.D. Thesis, University of Edinburgh.

Melia, K.M. (1987), *Learning and working: the occupational socialisation of student nurses*, Tavistock, London.

Melia, K.M. (1996), Personal communication.

Menzies, I.E.P. (1960), 'A case study in the functioning of social systems as a defence against anxiety', *Human Relations*, 13, 95-121.

Merton, R.K. (1967), 'The self-fulfilling prophecy', in, Coser, L.A. (ed, 1980) *The pleasures of sociology*, New English Library, London.

Milgram, S. (1963), 'Behavioral study of obedience', *Journal of Abnormal and Social Psychology*, 67, 371.

Morse, J.M. (1989), 'Gift-giving, reciprocity for care: gift giving in the patient nurse relationship', *Canadian Journal of Nursing Research*, 21, 1, 33-45.

Morse, J.M. and Johnson, J.L. (eds, 1991), *The illness experience: dimensions of suffering*, Sage, Newbury Park, California.

Moser, C.A. and Kalton, G. (1971), *Survey methods in social investigation*, 2nd Edition, Heinemann, London.

Navarro, V. (1976), *Medicine under capitalism*, London, Croom Helm.

Nursing Times (1992), 'Pioneer AIDS campaigner reveals he has illness and wins ovation', *Nursing Times*, 88, 45, 9.

Office of Population, Censuses and Surveys (OPCS, 1990), *Classification of occupations*, Her Majesty's Stationery Office, London.

Olesen, V.L. and Whittaker, E.W. (1967), *The silent dialogue*, Jossey Bass, San Francisco.

Orem, D. (1980), *Nursing: concepts of practice*, McGraw Hill, New York.

Orton, H.D. (1981), *Ward learning climate: the role of the ward sister in relation to student nurse learning on the ward*, Royal College of Nursing, London.

Papper, S. (1970), 'The undesirable patient', (editorial), *Journal of Chronic Diseases*, 22, 777-779.

Parker, R.S. (1990), 'Nurses' stories: the search for a relational ethic of care', *Advances in Nursing Science*, 13, 1, 31-40.

Parsons, T. (1951), *The social system*, Free Press, Glencoe Illinois.

Parsons, T. (1963), 'Power and the social system', in, Lukes, S. (ed, 1986) *Power,* Blackwell, Oxford.

Pembrey, S. (1979), 'Deference, authority, flirtation and stealth', *British Medical Journal,* 1st Dec., 1450-1451.

Pembrey, S. (1980), *The ward sister: key to nursing,* Royal College of Nursing, London.

Popper, K. (1959 revised 1968) *The logic of scientific discovery,* Hutchinson, London.

Porter, S. (1991), 'A participant observation study of power relationships between nurses and doctors in a general hospital', *Journal of Advanced Nursing,* 16, 6, 728-735.

Porter, S. (1993), 'Nursing research conventions: objectivity and obfuscation?', *Journal of Advanced Nursing,* 18, 137-143.

Psathas, G. (1968), 'The fate of idealism in nursing school', *Journal of Health and Social Behavior,* 9, 52-64.

Punch, M. (1986) *The politics and ethics of fieldwork,* Sage, California.

Quint, J.C. (1967), *The nurse and the dying patient,* Collier MacMillan, London.

Ragucci, A.T. (1972), 'The ethnographic approach in nursing research', *Nursing Research,* 21, 6, 485-490.

Reed, J. and Bond, S. (1991), 'Nurses' assessment of elderly patients in hospital', *International Journal of Nursing Studies,* 28, 1, 55-64.

Reinharz, S. (1992), *Feminist methods in social research,* Oxford University Press, New York.

Rex, J. (1961), 'Power, conflict, values and change', in, Worsley, P. (ed, 1978) *Modern sociology,* 2nd edition, Penguin, Harmondsworth.

Ritvo, M.M. (1963), 'Who are 'good' and 'bad' patients?', *The Modern Hospital,* 100, 6, 79-81.

Roberts, D. (1984), 'Non-verbal communication: popular and unpopular patients', in, Faulkner, A. (ed.) *Communication: recent advances in nursing series,* Churchill Livingstone, Edinburgh.

Roberts, H. (1992), 'Professionals' and parents' perceptions of A & E use in a children's' hospital', *The Sociological Review,* ,109-131.

Roper, N., Logan, W.W. and Tierney, A.J. (1980), *The elements of nursing,* Churchill Livingstone, Edinburgh.

Rosenhan, D.L. (1973), 'On being sane in insane places', *Science,* 179, 250-258.

Roth, J.A. (1962,a), 'The treatment of tuberculosis as a bargaining process', in, Rose, A.M. (ed, 1962) *Human behaviour and social processes: an interactional approach,* Routledge and Kegan Paul, London.

Roth, J. (1962,b), 'Comments on "secret observations" ', *Social Problems,* 9, 283-284.

Roth, J.A. (1972), 'Some contingencies of the moral evaluation and control of clientele', *American Journal of Sociology*, 77, 839.

Roy, C. (1980), 'The Roy adaptation model', in, Riehl, J.P. and Roy, C. (eds.) *Conceptual models for nursing practice*, Appleton Century Crofts, New York.

Royal College of Nursing (1977), *Ethics related to research in nursing*, Royal College of Nursing, London.

Rundell, S. (1991), 'A study of nurse patient interaction within a post-operative cardiothoracic high dependency unit', *Paper presented at Royal College of Nursing Research Advisory Group Conference*, University of Manchester, April.

Russell, B. (1938), 'The forms of power', in, Lukes, S. (Ed, 1986) *Power*, Blackwell, Oxford.

Salaman, G. (1986), *Working*, Tavistock, London.

Schatzman, L. and Strauss, A.L. (1973), *Field research: strategies for a natural sociology*, Prentice Hall, Englewood Cliffs, New Jersey.

Scheff, T.J. (1966), *Being mentally ill: a sociological theory*, Aldine, Chicago.

Schwartz, H. and Jacobs, J. (1979), *Qualitative sociology: a method to the madness*, New York, Free Press.

Silverman, D. (1975), *Qualitative methodology and sociology*, Gower, Aldershot.

Smart, P. (1985), *Michel Foucault*, Ellis Harwood and Tavistock, Chichester.

Smith, L. (1990), *A study of the help-seeking behaviours of alcohol-dependent and problem-drinking women*, Unpublished Ph.D. Thesis, University of Manchester.

Smith, P. (1992), *The emotional labour of nursing: how nurses care*, MacMillan, Basingstoke.

Spencer, G. (1982), 'Methodological issues in the study of bureaucratic elites: a case study of West Point', in, Burgess, R.G. (ed, 1982) *Field research: a sourcebook and field manual*, Allen and Unwin, London.

Stevens, B.J. (1979), *Nursing theory*, Little and Brown, Boston.

Steier, F. (ed, 1991), *Research and reflexivity*, Sage, London.

Stein, L. (1978), 'The doctor-nurse game', in, Dingwall, R. and McIntosh, J. (eds.) *Readings in the sociology of nursing*, Edinburgh, Churchill Livingstone.

Stern, P. (1985), 'Using grounded theory method in nursing research', in, Leininger, M.M. (ed.) *Qualitative research methods in nursing*, Grune and Stratton, Orlando.

Stockwell, F. (1972 reprinted 1984), *The unpopular patient*, Croom Helm, London.

Strauss, A., Schatzman, L., Ehrlich, D., Bucher, R. and Sabshin, M. (1963), 'The hospital and its negotiated order', in, Worsley, P. (ed, 1978) *Modern sociology*, 2nd edition, Penguin, Harmondsworth.

Strauss, A., Fagerhaugh, S., Suczek, B. and Wiener, C. (1982,a), 'The work of hospitalised patients', *Social Science and Medicine*, 16, 977-986.

Strauss, A., Fagerhaugh, S., Suczek, B. and Wiener, C. (1982,b), 'Sentimental work in the technologised hospital', *Sociology of Health and Illness*, 4, 3, 254-278.

Strauss, A.L. and Corbin, J. (1990), *Basics of qualitative research: grounded theory procedures and techniques*, Sage, Newbury Park.

Street, A.F. (1992), *Inside nursing: a critical ethnography of nursing practice*, State University of New York, Albany.

Strong, P.M. (1980), 'Doctors and dirty work: the case of alcoholism', *Sociology of Health and Illness*, 2, 1, 24-47.

Strong, P. and Robinson, J. (1990), *The NHS under new management*, Open University Press, Milton Keynes.

Tait, A.S. (1985), *Breast cancer and breast loss: some sociological considerations*, M.A. Thesis, University of Manchester.

Thompson, I.E., Melia, K.M. and Boyd, K.M. (1988) *Nursing ethics*, 2nd. edition, Churchill Livingstone, Edinburgh.

Tudor-Hart, J. (1975), 'The inverse care law', in, Cox, C. and Mead, A. (eds.) *A sociology of medical practice*, Collier MacMillan, London.

Turner, B.S. (1987), *Medical power and social knowledge*, Sage, London.

U.K.C.C. (1984, 1992), *Code of professional conduct for nurses, midwives and health visitors*, 2nd. edition, London, United Kingdom Central Council for Nursing, Midwifery and Health Visiting.

Waterworth, S. and Luker, K. (1990), 'Reluctant collaborators: do patients want to be involved in decisions concerning care?', *Journal of Advanced Nursing*, 15, 971-996.

Webb, C. (1984), 'Feminist methodology in nursing research', *Journal of Advanced Nursing*, 9, 3, 249-256.

Webb, C. (1987), 'Speaking up for advocacy', *Nursing Times*, 83, 34, 33-35.

Webb, C. (1989), 'Action research: philosophy, methods and personal experiences', *Journal of Advanced Nursing*, 14, 403-410.

Webb, C. (1992), 'The use of the first person in academic writing: objectivity, language and gatekeeping', *Journal of Advanced Nursing*, 17, 747-752.

Weber, M. (1947), *The theory of social and economic organisations*, translated by Parsons, T. (Ed), Free Press, New York.

Whyte, W.F. (1955), *Street corner society*, 2nd edition, University of Chicago Press, Chicago.

Wilkinson, S.M. (1991), *Factors influencing nurses' verbal communication with cancer patients*, Unpublished Ph.D. Thesis, University of Manchester.

Williams, A.M. (1989), *Interpreting an ethnography of nursing: exploring the boundaries of self, work and knowledge*, Unpublished Ph.D. Thesis, University of Manchester.

Williams, A. (1991), 'Practical ethics; interpretive processes in an ethnography of nursing', in, Aldridge, J., Griffiths, V. and Williams, A. (1991) *Rethinking; feminist research processes reconsidered*, Feminist Praxis: Studies in Sexual Politics No. 34, Manchester.

Williams, R. (1989), 'Awareness and control of dying: some paradoxical trends in public opinion', *Sociology of Health and Illness*, 11, 3. 201-212.

Williams, S. (1987), 'Goffman, interactionism, and the management of stigma in everyday life', in, Scambler, G. (ed, 1987) *Sociological theory and medical sociology*, Tavistock, London.

Wolf, Z.R. (1988), *Nurses' work: the sacred and the profane*, University Press, Pennsylvania.

Worsley, A. (1980), 'Exploration of student nurses' stereotypes of patients', *International Journal of Nursing Studies*, 17, 163-174.

Zborowski, M. (1952), 'Cultural components in response to pain', *Journal of Social Issues*, 8, 16-32.

Znaniecki, F. (1934), *The method of sociology*, Fanner and Rinehart, New York.

Index

207